Nursing Skills for Children and Young People's Mental Health

Laurence Baldwin

Editor

Nursing Skills for Children and Young People's Mental Health

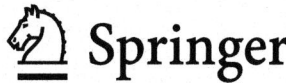 Springer

Editor
Laurence Baldwin
School of Nursing, Midwifery and Health
Coventry University
Coventry
Warwickshire
UK

ISBN 978-3-030-18678-4   ISBN 978-3-030-18679-1   (eBook)
https://doi.org/10.1007/978-3-030-18679-1

This Springer imprint is published by the registered company Springer Nature Switzerland AG
The registered company address is: Gewerbestrasse 11, 6330 Cham, Switzerland

This book is dedicated to all the children, young people and families I have worked with over the years, who have taught me so much about life and how to cope with what it throws at you.

My thanks to all the staff I have worked with in Nottingham, Mansfield and Derby CAMHS who have shared the journey, and who continue to work in very trying circumstances to deliver skilled help to those who need it.

To my mother, and late father, who always knew I would write a book (or part of one!) eventually.

And to my wife Katrina and my sons, Laurence, Luke and Lewis.

About the Book

This book focuses on what skills nurses have which are actually valued and needed by children and young people with mental health problems.

Whilst other books have focused on conditions, how they affect children and young people, and the treatments which can help, this book moves away from the formulaic pathway approach which has become popular in recent years and looks at what children and young people themselves have said they most value from those who seek to help them across the healthcare and other professions, and looks at why nursing skills are amongst the most valued things that our service users want from us. This focus on therapeutic relationships, establishing trusting, helpful ways of nursing and empowering children and young people to develop into healthy and resilient young adults has been neglected despite the feedback from those who need the help but often struggle to find it, or are wary of seeking help and reluctant to engage. It also stresses the importance of understanding the developmental and systemic context in which children and young people live their lives, and how this contributes to their needs.

Rather than focusing on different mental health conditions, this book will focus on the places where nurses encounter young people and how they use their skills to help them in that context. It will look at the role nurses play in specialist child and adolescent mental health settings (such as in-patient and community, as psychotherapists and on self-harm teams) and where paediatric nurses work with troubled young people (in emergency departments, paediatric wards and primary care). It will also look at a couple of areas, eating disorder services and consent-seeking, which benefit from nursing skills which are currently undervalued, but which should be seen as invaluable.

This focuses on what skills nurses have, but may not be consciously using, makes this book uniquely appealing to all nurses who work with children and young people with mental health problems, in whatever setting, and is aimed at both students and experienced professionals. The skills described, whilst central to nursing practice, are also useful for other professionals who have frontline contact with distressed children and young people, such as allied health professionals, social workers, teachers and third sector staff.

Contents

About the Editor

Laurence Baldwin spent over 30 years in the NHS working mostly in specialist Child and Adolescent Mental Health Services, for the last 13 years as a Nurse Consultant. During this time, he also became an independent nurse prescriber and represented the Royal College of Nursing at various national forums, including the CAMHS Taskforce that developed the 'Future in Mind' policy. Clinically he has interests in ADHD, Autistic Spectrum Disorders, and self-harm, as well as developing service-user led research projects. His PhD was on professional identity in CAMHS, and he is now an Assistant Professor in Mental Health Nursing at Coventry University where he leads on research methodology at postgraduate level and has recently developed an online module for the MSc Nursing.

Contributors

Marie Armstrong Hopewood, Nottinghamshire Healthcare NHS Foundation Trust, Nottingham, UK

Laurence Baldwin School of Nursing, Midwifery and Health, Coventry University, Coventry, Warwickshire, UK

Ann Marie Cox North Staffordshire Combined NHS Trust, North Staffordshire, UK

Moira Goodman Retired, formerly Nottinghamshire Healthcare NHS Foundation Trust, Nottingham, UK

Stephanie Mansfield School of Nursing, Midwifery and Health, Coventry University, Coventry, Warwickshire, UK

Tim McDougall Greater Manchester Mental Health NHS Foundation Trust, Manchester, UK

Gemma Robbins School of Nursing, Midwifery and Health, Coventry University, Coventry, Warwickshire, UK

Children and Young People's Nursing, Coventry University, Coventry, Warwickshire, UK

Katrina Singhatey Cognitive Behavioural Psychotherapist (Private Practice), Nottingham, UK

Leanne Walker Derbyshire Healthcare NHS Foundation Trust, Derbyshire, UK

Chapter 1
What Nursing Skills Are We Using with Children and Young People Who Experience Mental Health Difficulties?

Laurence Baldwin

1.1 Introduction

This book is about nursing skills, a rather vague and undervalued term. Over the years, I have come to the conclusion that nursing does not really have a set of skills which ONLY nurses can do, but it does have a set of skills which it prizes much more highly than other professions, and which comprise a distinctive approach to helping others. It is this set of skills, on which this book will be focusing, and showing, I hope, how nursing does have a unique contribution to the mental health and well-being of children, young people, and their families. Implicit in this approach is a recognition that all of the skills we will be looking at and discussing are actually used as well by other professionals, such as teachers, social workers, psychologists, psychiatrists, and counsellors. But none of those professional trainings stress the importance of these skills as being central to the work; usually they have another core underlying belief which is central to their way of working. The skills we will be discussing, and the importance nurses attach to them, are what makes a nursing skills approach distinctly important and unique. I hope we can also demonstrate that these skills, and this nursing skills approach, match up very well with what children and young people actually prize most highly in the people from whom they seek help when they are in emotional distress. In that sense, I hope this book will be of use to other professionals as well as to nurses, who are in regular contact with distressed young people of all sorts.

L. Baldwin (✉)
School of Nursing, Midwifery and Health, Coventry University, Coventry, Warwickshire, UK
e-mail: ac1273@coventry.ac.uk

© Springer Nature Switzerland AG 2020
L. Baldwin (ed.), *Nursing Skills for Children and Young People's Mental Health*,
https://doi.org/10.1007/978-3-030-18679-1_1

1

1.2   Background to Nursing Fields in the UK, and Their Distinctive Approaches

Nursing is a very 'broad church' with a lot of variations and ways of enacting the central essence of being a nurse. This book will concentrate on its enactment in the United Kingdom, but will make reference to how nursing is done in the rest of the world. Unique to the UK is the separation of training into four 'fields', so nurses train in either 'adult nursing', 'children and young people's nursing', 'mental health nursing', or 'learning disabilities nursing' (sometimes called 'intellectual disabilities nursing'). Whilst these four fields have much in common, and in university settings much of the core curriculum is delivered together, they remain distinct from each other. This allows specialisation at a much earlier stage than in other countries, where psychiatric nursing, for example, becomes a postgraduate training, and what the UK regards as 'adult nursing' is the first-level training for every nurse. But it also means that there are gaps in knowledge, so specialist CAMH nurses may be trained in any of the above fields initially and therefore have a skew to their knowledge. Historically, most CAMHS specialists came from mental health nursing, but that training does not generally focus on children and young people's mental health, it spends a great deal of time on how mental health issues manifest themselves in working age and older adults, because historically that is where services have focussed, and where the demand has been for nursing skills (in adult mental health inpatient and community services). Likewise, children and young people's nursing has focussed on the physical health of its age specialisation, and how this manifests itself differently from physical health needs in adults. Traditionally, it has relatively little emphasis on the emotional well-being of young people and on mental health, although for both these fields of training this has been improving recently as more awareness of children and young people's emotional needs has improved. Learning disabilities nursing covers the lifespan much better, given that intellectual disabilities are lifelong conditions, and does have some emphasis on the comorbid mental health conditions which can develop in this group of people, but it is only relatively recently that these transferrable skills have been recognised as being important for CAMHS provision.

One way of illustrating this gap into which CAMH nursing has fallen is to look at how the textbooks for these fields deal with children and young people's mental health. A recent series by Sage Publications released textbooks on mental health nursing (Wright and McKeown 2018) and children and young people's nursing (Price and McAlinden 2017), both take a fairly standard approach to textbook production, which reflects how nursing is taught in the UK. The volume on mental health nursing has chapters on eating disorders (which generally start before the age of 18), which mention aetiology and treatment in younger people, and a chapter on child and adolescent care, with 27 pages from a total of 712 pages. The volume on children and young people's nursing likewise has a chapters on care of the child or young person with mental health problems (which is 15 pages long), and three chapters on communicating with children and the development of emotions and well-being issues. If we include these, we get a total of 61 pages out of a total of 688 pages. Both of these books are excellent textbooks, and I use each of them in the teaching I do on undergraduate and specialist courses at my home university, but this disparity illustrates well the way both fields of nursing seem, historically, to treat children and young people's mental health problems as an SEP—'Someone Else's Problem' (Adams 1982).

Specialist CAMH nursing has, therefore, long been seen as an orphaned discipline, and as 'someone else's problem', belonging neither fully to mental health nor to children's nursing. In some ways, it has also been seen very much as a speciality, despite longstanding efforts to see children and young people's mental health and well-being as 'everybody's business' (MHF 1999). The nursing training routes in the UK which have neglected this area, by concentrating on what they see as their core business, have contributed to this, and the same is true for other disciplines. Clinical psychology has done better in this respect, and has always had a focus on children's developmental psychology from an early age (Faulconbridge et al. 2018), so their training does tend to emphasise this area well, but they remain a relatively small discipline, though very influential in policy and service development terms. Social work has vacillated between a generic and more specialist focus in its training (Pierson 2011), and has a historic influence through the child guidance movement, which preceded current CAMHS provision. Its present focus, however, within the area of children's care, is primarily on safeguarding and protecting children, and within this field has a particular approach that focusses on physical abuse and sexual abuse, with a more difficult relationship when dealing with neglect and emotional abuse. Medical psychiatry has a strong emphasis on the medical model of understanding mental health and illness, despite a long tradition within the speciality of child and adolescent psychiatry of a sociological perspective on the understanding of children and young people's needs. Psychiatrists in the UK are medically trained doctors first and then specialise in psychiatry, with at least one placement with younger people, but it does struggle to recruit into the CAMHS posts (BMJ 2016). Amongst the Allied Health Professions, the most prominent group working regularly in this area is Occupational Therapy, which brings its own central perspective of the value of meaningful activity (either in employment, education, or other forms of purposeful activity) to the mental health needs of this group (RCOT 2019). These are very broad brush descriptions of the central preoccupations of other professional groups and apologies are due for some inevitable level of stereotyping. Each of these professional groups will employ the sort of skills which we are going to look at as being central to a nursing approach, and some individuals within each professional group will give these skills prominence and deliver them very well, but they are not core to the professional training, in the same way as they are to nursing. The underlying philosophy of each profession is often buried so deep into those who practice that they become part of their identity and lose the ability to verbalise those 'taken-for-granted' ways of working, which are central to their identity (Baldwin 2008).

1.3   What Makes Nursing Distinctive in Its Approach to Working with CYP?

In order to look at the emphasis of different professional groups and tease out the distinctiveness of nursing strengths in CAMHS, we need to go beyond the current political context and look little more deeply. There is, of course, a huge body of literature relating to the theory and conceptual frameworks that different professions bring to the task of providing care or therapy. This often relates to the broader context of the parent profession for those groups, who have wider professional allegiances; the history and development of physical health nursing is very different to that of mental health nursing. So, whilst, for example, mental health nursing usually benefits from the positive press that nursing enjoys (despite the Mid-Staffordshire tragedy) its evolution has differed over the years. Nolan's (1993) history shows how adult mental health nursing moved from asylum-based care to its present format, and CAMH nursing has followed on the back of those changes. It is important to look at what constitutes a particular intervention, particularly within mental health teams, to see if there is anything distinctive about those interventions that can be seen to add value beyond the application of a set of skills and competences. There are several different professional groups working within mental health teams and CAMHS as we have seen. For some, the conceptual framework in which they work pertains purely to mental health work. Psychology and the psychotherapies fall within this group, even where they are applied to physical healthcare, whilst other professional groups come from a wider umbrella, forming only a subgroup of the wider profession. These groups follow often quite divergent paths from their parent professional body and the specialisation into mental health, and for our purposes into child mental health, which gives a degree of distance from those parent bodies. Psychiatrists (and specialist Child and Adolescent Psychiatrists), for example, work in a way that is connected to, but distant from, the work of many other medical doctors. Allied Health Professionals in mental health, such as Occupational Therapists, are also seen only as a subgroup of their main profession, and a dietician in a mental health trust will work with a very different client group to a dietician in a physical healthcare setting.

This distinction can also be drawn for social workers and nurses. Yet all of these professional groups retain links to their parent group and need to conform to the professional regulation and governance of those groups. The identity of 'nurse' compared to 'mental health nurse' is one of conflict, for arguably a mental health nurse has more in common with other staff in mental health services in terms of skills and competences than they do with most physical healthcare nurses, yet they retain a nursing identity. Nursing, and particularly nursing within CAMHS, therefore faces a challenge of identity in that it is distant from its parent group, and in many ways shares more in common with the other members of the mental health team, including the social workers and psychotherapists, than it does with other nurses. During my career this has become very stark at times. As a Nurse Consultant, for example, I was part of my Trust's senior nursing team looking at minimum standards for nursing competencies, and had to resist the directive that all nurses would be doing refresher training in performing injections. This seems a sensible safety feature except that injections are not a routine part of a community CAMHS nurses work (parents administer medications, and we generally do not use any injectable medications), so the last injection I administered as a nurse was in 1989!

1.4   The Development of Adult Mental Health Nursing

Nolan (ibid) traces current mental health nursing practice primarily back to the asylums and the initial role of attendants, who were largely subservient to the medical profession in the treatment of the insane. In fact there is a longer history of the mentally disturbed being humanely treated through the more enlightened monastic and religious houses, to which he alludes in his references to Bethlem Hospital and its predecessors. This function, along with the mainstream healing and hospital facilities provided within religious organisations, failed, he contends, to cope with the expansion of population that the Industrial Revolution brought to this country. The expanded unmet needs led to the establishment of asylums. Indeed, there remains a link between the religious vocation and secular caring through mental health nursing and other caring professions (Crawford et al. 1998).

In the modern era, however, Hildegard Peplau is largely credited with focussing psychiatric nursing on the therapeutic relationship between the nurse and the person they are nursing. In the early 1960s (article reproduced in Peplau 1982), she was looking at this in relation to nursing people with schizophrenia, and much psychiatric and mental health nursing theory has developed from this approach. In the UK, Annie Altschul (Tilley 1999) brought many of Peplau's ideas across the Atlantic and translated them into a British context, adding her own distinctive element by emphasizing the 'common sense' approach as being a particularly nursing contribution. In the same tradition, Professor Phil Barker and others in Newcastle have explored ideas about what is the 'proper focus' of psychiatric nursing (explicitly drawing on Peplau's work), and the reasons people might need psychiatric nurses (Barker et al. 1995, 1999). Barker's main thesis is that, while 'caring' is often seen within wider nursing as a core element, there does not exist an adequate definition of 'caring'. He feels that, whilst there is no harm in nurses identifying what caring means to them, this could not, however, become the 'raison d'étre' of nursing. Barker points out that if caring is the essence of nursing, not only must all nursing involve caring, but that caring must only occur in nursing, or occur in some unique way. This is clearly not the case. He concludes that if nursing is to be defined, globally, by any one thing, it is the social construction of the nurse's role. The nurse's role changes more as a function of societal shifts than as a result of any actualisation of the 'essential' nature of the profession. Barker has been scathing about the 'nursing theology' of nursing as caring, and religious overtones of nursing apologists like Watson (1985). Professor Barker (1999) noted, for example, that many of Watson's defining features of nursing can also be found in the psychotherapy literature, when the nature and role of psychotherapy are described. Barker concludes with the important point that, as long as nursing is defined in terms of what nurses do, rather than what nursing is meant to achieve, an evaluation of its worth will be impossible, however its 'core' is defined.

This is an important point, as much of the literature relating to 'role' within nursing does restrict itself to a description of function. Duffy and Lee (1998), for example, make good points about role ambiguity, but essentially describe the way the nurses work, rather than analysing that work in the context of a theoretical or conceptual framework. This phenomenon also occurs in one of the few pieces of work specifically on CAMH nursing (Leighton et al. 2001). Repper (2000) sees the difficulty in defining mental health nursing as springing from the variety of roles inherent in this field of nursing. She notes the essential difficulty of measuring the nature of nursing, compared to the move toward quantifiable evidence-based approaches to service delivery as originally espoused by Gournay (1995). Her solution is to recognise the multiplicity and diversity of nursing roles, whilst reinforcing that service users' value nurses for their 'ordinariness'. In particular, she recognises that each nurse will bring individual skills that will be used in different ways with different situations and relating differently to a variety of service user needs. An early study of the general public by Walker et al. (1998) emphasised that those members of the public who had any knowledge or opinion on the role of mental health nurses valued them primarily for caring, talking and listening. Pilgrim and Rogers (1994) had also found that service users valued 'ordinariness' and the basic listening skills demonstrated by nurses. They also found that having enough time to employ these skills was directly (and inversely) related to the grade of the staff, so non-qualified staff and student nurses were the most valued, at least in a ward setting, because they were the most available. There is also an implication that this 'ordinariness' relates to either a lack of expertise, or consciously adopting a non-expert stance, in contrast to other professionals. The extreme conclusion of this would be that rather than training people, the solution is simply to recruit the right sort of intuitive staff in the first place. Others have attempted to quantify which human qualities can be recognised and enhanced in order to understand the process that allows good nursing. Graham (2001), for example cited holism, partnership and empowerment alongside relationship-building, as essential elements of the meaning of nursing. The conscious employment of skills, and an active use of self-awareness, rather than relying on intuitive or innate qualities, seems, therefore, to contribute towards an understanding of the essence of mental health nursing.

In 'Working in Partnership' (DH 1994), it was suggested that psychiatric nursing '…should play a central role in the provision of high quality mental health care.' Yet defining what nursing has to offer, and what nurses actually do, or ought to be doing, remains a contentious and difficult area, even in adult mental health settings. The Chief Nursing Officer's review of mental health nursing specifically asked for views on the core values and roles of mental health nursing (DH 2005), yet when that review was published (DH 2006), it held back from defining which values actually underpinned mental health nursing specifically. It referred instead to more generic principles such as the Recovery Approach and the need to (p13): '…move away from a traditional model of care to a biopsychosocial and values-based approach.' The review was called 'From Values to Actions', yet the values listed are not specifically nursing values; they are based on the wider principles of service user's need. This is in itself laudable, but does not help in defining the perspective of nursing in any way that might differentiate it from other mental health professions, who also aspire to utilise these general principles. In defining a conceptual framework, or even an underlying set of specifically nursing values, the review is therefore unhelpful. It concentrates instead on the actions, with only Recommendation 5 (of 17) being suggestive of a specifically nursing approach to the task. Recommendation 5 (p29) is that: 'All MHNs will be able to develop strong therapeutic relationships with service users and carers.' Again the influence of Peplau and her followers is evident here. Other recommendations, such as the importance of holistic assessments (Recommendation 6) might be indicative of a values based approach, but are harder to define as specifically nursing approaches as many other professional groups espouse holism as important (whilst none have the same emphasis on therapeutic relationship building as central to their approach).

Duffy and Lee (ibid) suggested that there remains a dilemma for many nurses in practice between the 'clinical support role', of running the ward, administering medication and completing necessary paperwork, and the development of 'specialist clinician' roles. They suggest that nurses are often tolerant of role ambiguity, and would be happy to develop either or both directions for the future role of nursing. However, they also warn that many of the 'clinical support' roles could be fulfilled by people who are not trained nurses. The previous Department of Health (1994) review of mental health nursing 'Working in Partnership' had also struggled with precisely defining the unique role of mental health nurses. The movement towards looking at what you actually need nurses for, and which of their functions could be fulfilled by others, is also prevalent in some influential areas of policy making. The Sainsbury Centre (1997) published ideas about the increased use of 'generic workers' with relevant experience, and was based on skill mix concepts. Their report focused primarily on the needs of those with more severe and enduring mental health problems (and does not mention CAMHS). They note, however, that the role of nurses is often differentiated from other disciplines as 'caring, rehabilitation, and medication supervision skills'. However the report, whilst addressing the training needs of various professionals within the multi-disciplinary teams who currently provide adult mental health care, suggest a focus on establishing core competences and standards for all workers. The report affirms the genericism of mental health work, with each specialist discipline having a specific contribution to make on top of the generic element of the work. What it fails to suggest is what those specialist contributions might be, beyond nursing being a 'caring' profession. Other professions would claim 'caring' as a useful addition (though sometimes with a warning about professional boundaries), but not put it at the centre of their philosophy. The Sainsbury Centre has led in this with the Capable Practitioner document (Sainsbury Centre 2001).

The Sainsbury Centre had begun this push towards the genericisation of skills when it published a report on the working of Community Mental Health Teams (Onyett et al. 1995), which looked at the roles, relationships, and job satisfaction of team members in terms of core profession. It also specifically excluded from its study teams for older people, alcohol and drugs misuse and learning difficulties. The report does not seem to recognise the existence of CAMHS (neither excluding nor including them, simply omitting any reference to them). Many of the issues they report (p21), however, are very familiar to professionals in CAMHS, particularly the 'special dilemma' of being members of, and having loyalty to, both discipline and team. These difficulties are defined as being torn between the egalitarianism inherent in the aims of the community mental health movement, with its associated role blurring, and the desire to maintain traditional, socially valued role definitions and practices. They felt that ideal conditions would be for each discipline to have a clear and valued role within the team, and that the team as a whole has a clear role. With regard to nurses, the report makes some curiously conflicting conclusions. Nurses are seen as an essential element of Community Mental Health Teams, being present in 93% of them, but are amongst the most exhausted, with the least satisfaction about their work relationships. However, they are also reported to be the members of the team with the highest team identification and professional identification. They are described as having a high degree of clarity about the role of the team and their own role within the team, which was previously noted as 'ideal conditions' for working in such a team. The report does not expand on what these nurses saw as being their role, or how it differed from that of the other disciplines.

What this demonstrates, then, is the difficulty of nurses in mental health in articulating what they bring by virtue of their professional background and training, to the task. This in turn opens up the question of whether that is important, or if, as the Sainsbury Centre reports suggest, this is no longer relevant, as long as the task is completed.

1.5   The Evolution of Child and Adolescent Mental Health Nursing

Within CAMHS, there is very poor documentation and very little published about the development of services. Whilst there are many academic papers on child development and specific syndromes, and a large body of literature on the individual therapies used, the development of services and the contribution of different disciplines to service delivery have not been extensively recorded. CAMH nursing has always seen itself as a 'Cinderella service', being a speciality within a speciality, and falling between two camps, i.e., neither truly belonging to mental health nor to paediatrics. Nurses have been involved in caring for children and young people with mental health problems since the 1960s, but have only in the last 25 years been involved in their outpatient care. The use of nurses on inpatient units is easier to understand in terms of traditional nursing skills. Direct care on wards was a natural place for nurses to have input as child psychiatry units developed in the UK. Child and adolescent psychiatric inpatient units were developed in the 1960s and 1970s following a Ministry of Health Memorandum of 1964 (cited in Horrocks 1986). Haldane (1963) first looked at the 'functions' of a nurse on such a unit, from a medical point of view. This concentrated on what would now be called 'milieu therapy', the establishing of an environment conducive to change, and the development of therapeutic relationships between children and the nurses (i.e. Geanellos 1999). Much of what Haldane (ibid) describes could be seen as a substitute parenting function for children whose parents were not present on the wards. Even at this stage, however, a need for flexibility amongst the nursing staff is stressed, and he made a point of saying that the nurses required on these units needed slightly different qualities to those employed on adult wards. It is worth noting that this is a medical point of view and there is no credit for any nursing input into the preparation of the article. When Haldane et al. (1971) later revisited this subject, he laid more stress on the part played by nurses in the psychotherapeutic work of the unit. The way nurses were involved in running therapeutic group work was becoming much more established, whilst the intensity and depth of the relationships developed between nursing staff and the young people were again noted to be very important.

Although not specifically mentioned, this seems to reflect the influence of Peplau and Altschul on psychiatric nursing in this period, as noted before. Haldane at this point attempted to define the levels of nursing skills. He defined 'basic nursing skills' in this context as the parental caring function. 'Special nursing skills' are seen as more sophisticated self-awareness, with greater technical skills, and an understanding of psychodynamic processes. This would equate with mental health skills in other areas. He then goes on to define 'advanced nursing skills' as more in-depth analytical understanding, and 'consultant nursing skills', which include training (of others) and independent practice development. Haldane justifies the use of nurses instead of a proposed 'generic care worker' on the grounds of nurses' knowledge of organic and psychosomatic illness, psychopharmacology, and 'technical nursing procedures'. This is an early attempt to differentiate nursing skills from those of other workers, and it is important to note that as these are not 24 hour care skills, they are transferable to outpatient settings. It is also the first instance of the medical model of nurse training being highlighted as a valuable (at least to medical staff) asset not available from other staff groups. At that point in time, however, he did not see a role for nurses working outside of an institutional setting. His analysis of nursing skills in CAMH seems to rely for a conceptual framework on physical caring, mental health skills and the therapeutic use of self in the development of therapeutic relationships. Subsequently, what was written in the 1980s and 1990s about the overall theory and practice of child and adolescent mental health nursing (e.g. Delaney 1992; Puskar et al. 1990; Hogarth 1991), continued to see the work of CAMH nurses as primarily institutionally based. Wilkinson (1983) noted that it was 'rare' to find nursing totally in the community, whilst Bhoyrub and Morton (1983) state that nurses are not integral to the outpatient child psychiatry clinic, and described the nursing task in outpatient settings, which seemed to consist of greeting the patients and preparing them to meet their therapist. By the mid 1980s, the report 'Bridges Over Troubled Waters' (Horrocks 1986) was published, looking at the specific needs of adolescents. This had an effect mostly on the provision of adolescent inpatient services, but it does make some comments about nursing roles. Its recommendations (p68) include the idea that:

...each profession should define its own role in the management of disturbance in adolescence, and state what it can contribute to the work of others.

Earlier the report had looked at the differing roles within the treatment of adolescents. It emphasized the broader recommendation by stating (p61):

The nursing profession needs to define the specialist contribution which nurses can make to the care and treatment of adolescents with specific psychiatric disorder.

It also noted that nurses must work increasingly in community settings, either as specialist Community Psychiatric Nurses (CPNs), or in an outreach function from inpatient units. The definition of what specialist contribution nurses made, which was different from other professions, was not made explicit in the report. Role definition was, however, touched on in a section discussing levels of staffing and training needs (p12–14). Here mention is made of nurses' increasing work with families rather than individual patients on units, and of nurses' developing ability to offer specific interventions for specific problems. It also notes the increasing number of nurses working in child guidance clinics. In this section, it identifies the specific ability of nurses to offer:

...close and continuing support and therapy, enhanced by knowledge of the patient.

In the community, nurses were seen as offering support, advice and consultation to a variety of agencies, although again this would also reflect what other team members in CAMHS would be able to provide. Given that the historical evidence for nurses moving out of inpatient units is very poorly documented (Baldwin 2002), this is one of the few clues evident about the reason for nursing staff joining outpatient teams, which were often initially attached to inpatient units to provide continuity of care.

Usually, the Consultant Child Psychiatrist running the unit would also have responsibility for outpatient care, and could see some benefit of using experienced nursing staff in that area of work too. The most experienced nurses, who had developed family work skills from within their inpatient work, were seconded to the outpatient teams, where their jobs later became permanent, and the nursing workforce later expanded. In the same year as 'Bridges Over Troubled Waters' (ibid) was published Professor Rutter, the leading UK child and adolescent psychiatrist at the time, made a series of predictions for the next 30 years in child psychiatry (Rutter 1986). He suggested that there was likely to be an increase in the development of a course to produce nurses, who could act as independent clinicians. This move for nurses toward independent practice within the community he saw as based on the social work model, with a need to change the salary and status hierarchy to reward clinical nurses. He also stressed the need for clinical research and teaching to be integrated within the care functions of nursing, as is now explicitly the case for Consultant Nurses, and increasingly for Clinical Nurse Specialists and Advanced

Nurse Practitioners. This illustrates some concurrence at the time in the thinking of how nursing roles might be developed. He did not, however, cover the issue of what the profession actually brought by way of an underlying conceptual framework.

1.6   The Expansion of Roles in Child and Adolescent Mental Health Nursing

Within the British literature, the earliest reference to nursing roles in community CAMHS is McMorrow (1990). He noted the proliferation of job titles in CAMHS and suggested that this reflects the uncertainty as to exactly what role nurses were meant to perform when those posts had been set up. A clearer role, he felt, might have brought with it more uniformity of job title across different services. Limerick and Baldwin (2000) later discussed some of these issues in terms of generic workers and core skills for CAMHS staff. They made the point that professional account-ability is important in an era when the move towards generic workers tends to emphasise capabilities over training. Other writers have made efforts to define the nursing contribution but these are often incidental to the central thesis of their argu-ment. Lacey (1999), for example, refers to child mental health nurses as making good Primary Mental Health Workers (PMHWs) because of their holistic approach, good interpersonal skills and communication skills. She noted that in her survey, a high proportion of PMHWs at that time had a nursing background, and the holism of nurse training led to an integrative approach to their work. Similarly Leighton et al. (2001), whilst aiming to provide a detailed profile of the nursing contribution within outpatient CAMHS do not explicitly address areas of difference from their non-nursing colleagues. They offer a good description of function and skills likely to be employed, with emphasis on therapeutic relationships, assessment and treat-ment modalities, and a discussion of the limitations imposed on CAMH nurses. They conclude that nurses' lack of specialism, whilst in many ways a strength, also prevented CAMH nurses from promoting the work they did. This links to the con-cept that nurses make good generic workers within CAMHS, in this case described as eclecticism, rather than having areas of distinctive expertise or strength. In more general articles about children's mental health needs, the applicability of nursing skills is also mentioned. Townley (2002), for example, comments on a wide range of areas where nurses have an opportunity to promote good mental health, but does not specify how nursing skills specifically would be used. He implies that nurses' communication skills would enable them to engage with children and young people but he does not spell this out. Likewise Davies et al. (2002), commenting on the CAMH service in South Wales, make passing reference to nurses employed as ther-apists, rather than with a nursing job title, but do not enlarge or comment on this. The implication is that nurses may be under-represented in the workforce calcula-tions because they are not all employed in a specific nursing capacity, but rather for their generic skills, with a generic job title.

One of the few pieces of work that made a concerted effort to define the nursing role in the developing CAMHS agenda remains unpublished. Sue Croom's secondment to the Department of Health led to a draft report, which was never widely circulated (Croom 2001). Her key point (para 6) was that:

Skilled nursing involves working closely with children and families to anticipate needs, to support, to nurture and to provide key therapeutic interventions. Yet because it is sustained as a continuous and seamless process its complexity can be invisible to some observers who assume that it is a less sophisticated activity than it actually is. Skilled nursing is crucial to a modern CAMH service and needs to be strengthened and developed.

Much of the rest of her report was taken up in the preparatory work ahead of the publication of the NSF for Children (2004). This included suggestions for strengthening nurse education and the need to recognise the contribution of primary care nurses in the continuum of CAMH nursing (Baldwin 2005).

As nursing has established itself within CAMHS, there have also been further attempts to provide up to date textbooks on CAMHS care in the community. Dhogra et al. (2001) concentrated on primary care and the range of interventions available. In addressing primary care, there was an overview of treatment approaches available and no real attempt was made to relate these to underlying conceptual frameworks of different professional groups. McDougall (2006) did address specifically nursing approaches, at least in the title, though this is not evident in all the chapters of the book itself. There is again an attempt to describe the range of different approaches and treatments in which CAMH nurses are currently involved. These chapters are largely descriptive, however, and there is little attempt to look at what conceptual frameworks underpin the nursing application of these approaches.

Two international studies have made efforts to look at aspects of inpatient CAMH nursing. These are important in that they relate to the nursing role in community CAMHS. Scharer (1999) took a grounded theory approach in the USA to uncover ideas about relationship building by nurses, and did relate these skills to core nursing skills. She noted that nurses were in the best position to develop relationships with parents of young people accommodated on the inpatient unit. She focussed on this because nurses often saw the parents at times of stress, i.e., when collecting or returning their children to the unit. Scharer felt the intensity of this experience led to much quicker and more accurate relationships between nurses and the parents than they might have with other staff members who saw them at different, more settled, times. Rene Geanellos, in an Australian context, put emphasis on the nurse's ability to create a therapeutic milieu within the CAMH in patient unit (Geanellos 1999). Her study concentrates on the nursing skills used during time spent with young people on the unit, and the human qualities used by nurses over the lengthy periods of time they spend on shift. She does, however, point out that despite the fact that nurses are most likely to be the ones using milieu theory, nurses are rarely generating nurse-based theory to support their work.

In the arena of outpatient or community CAMHS in England, there remains little published that is specific. Only one previous study attempts to address this issue in any depth (Baldwin 2002). This study covered six different English CAMH services, and did make attempts to look at perceptions of nursing roles within these teams. When respondents were asked what they knew of the history of the introduction of nurses into these teams, there was an overall recognition that the nursing posts were never clearly planned, as we have inferred earlier in this chapter. Within this study there was, however, a perception (proposed by disciplines other than nurses and doctors) that nurses were in the teams because they are more compliant to doctors orders than other disciplinary groups, being more used to working within a medical hierarchical model. The study developed a detailed series of themes within the interviews that were carried out:

- Team composition and history. Although each team visited had a generally similar task their composition varied quite considerably;
- The strength of clinical autonomy within CAMHS. All the nurses interviewed fulfilled the criteria for autonomous practice suggested by Leddy and Pepper (1993);
- Clarity of specific roles of non-nursing staff in CAMHS. Most of the interviewees were able to identify clear differentiated roles and methods of working for the non-nursing disciplines within the teams. It was also recognised that all members of CAMHS (including the nurses) had a generic core function, which overlapped and in which differences of practice were much less marked;
- Difficulty in defining the nursing role. Interviewees found it much more difficult to define the core, defining role of the nursing staff. Although several nursing skills were mentioned by different interviewees, there was no consensus at all as to what nurses brought to the team by virtue of their nurse training and experience.
- Perhaps, the most worrying aspect was that nurses were taken 'for granted'. Their role was assumed, although not well-defined;
- Personality versus professional training. In teams where there was more than one nurse, it was acknowledged that the different nurses did their jobs in often very different ways, largely dependent on their character;
- The generic function and role overlaps. It was clear that the generic function, which all team members fulfilled in addition to any specialist function that they have, was a function performed well by nurses.

Whilst this study remains the only detailed published examination of roles in CAMH nursing, it has a number of methodological limitations. It was limited to a small convenience sample, and lacked a sound academic theory or philosophical underpinning on which to base its analysis, confining itself to a simple thematic analysis.

1.7   Other Aspects of Nursing Applied to CAMH Care

If Geanellos (ibid) put an emphasis on therapeutic milieu, alongside therapeutic relationships, it is worth looking a bit more at how nurses have traditionally created the conditions for people to get better as a fundamental of care. The earliest nurse theory concentrated on improving environment, including instilling hope and saw creating conditions for the body to heal itself as the essence of the nursing process (Nightingale 1859). This 'environmental theory' of nursing also has a focus on individualized care and the relationship that develops between nurse and patient. Nightingale envisioned nurses being present with their patients almost all of the time, (the vocational element was strong in those days) and even addresses instructions for what others should do in the nurses' absence, which foreshadows another invisible element of nursing, that of 'being there'. Allan's (2002) ethnographic study of an outpatient fertility clinic noted that both nurses and patients put value on the physical presence of nurses, even if they could not identify what it was they were doing except providing comfort by what she calls 'hovering'. Whilst this was not a mental health example, the observations are understood in a psychological sense, and are noted as being part of a function that is invisible and hard to define but which has value for patients, even if it is very difficult to ascribe a metric to that value. Inpatient care has more obvious application of this presence that nurses provide, as the only group of staff are with patients constantly. Other groups, medical doctors, for example, may be available around the clock, but their interactions with patients are limited to usually short encounters with a specific purpose. This may be true also of nursing staff on the ward that their face-to-face encounters during a shift with individuals may be short or task-focussed, but those same staffs remain physically present on the ward, essentially for the whole eight or twelve hours. In her recent book, Molly Case (2019) also talks about this presence issue, and the way that nurses (in her case cardiac nurses) provide a continuity of care over lengthy shifts and several days, so that patients appreciate the familiarity and comfort of the same people being around them in a way that other professionals are often not.

During that time as well nursing staff, in particular mental health nursing staff, need to maintain some kind of therapeutic relationship with each individual even during very stressful times. They need to keep this relationship effective even if they are not able to immediately meet the patients' wishes or their perceived needs. In extreme circumstances, mental health nurses may be involved in a restraint situation, involved in rapid tranquilisation, or close observations with highly disturbed individuals, yet still need to be around to maintain care after other staff have left the situation. This intensity of relationship over a sustained period of time requires nurses to develop ways of 'being there' through the good times and the bad. This fits with what we have previously discussed in the approach of Peplau and others.

Naturally, simple physical presence is not enough, 'availability' in a therapeutic sense needs also to be signalled and enacted, and the presence needs to be useful, so issues of compassion, which again used to be taken for granted as being a part of a nursing presence, have been highlighted in the work of Paul Gilbert in developing compassion-focussed therapies (Gilbert 2005), and applied to mental health nursing by Stickley and Spandler (2014). This has been specifically applied to CAMH nursing in a relatively unknown book by Fitzgibbon and Holyoake (2002 p50–51), which ascribes the link between 'being there' and caring to Appleton (1993) but sees this enacted in the comforting role previously noted by Haldane (ibid). They go on to emphasize the uniqueness of this role to the nursing profession among the others, and link it to both containment of distress and taking a holistic caring viewpoint to the provision of what young people need whilst in distress.

1.8   Nurse Consultant, Non-medical/Independent Prescribing and Responsible Clinician Roles

Another development, which has further served to blur the lines between disciplines, and increase the genericism within CAMHS has been the development of expanded and primarily quasi-medical roles for nurses. In many ways, this is a natural extension of the increasing levels of autonomy which nurses have been encouraged to take on or have pushed for themselves. Starting in the early 2000s, CAMHS was quick to adopt the Nurse Consultant role for its most experienced nurses (McDougall 2005), and push forward the advanced level of autonomous practice that this gave them. Either as specialists in particular areas, such as ADHD (Ryan and McDougall 2008) or self-harm (McDougall et al. 2010), or as generic lead nurse roles within outpatient services, the ability to develop nursing practice over a range of practice areas was seized on and used to further independent and autonomous practice. As non-medical and independent prescribing became more widespread, it has also been a natural move for some nurses within CAMHS, either as part of their Nurse Consultant role, or as a distinct role to undertake the course in independent prescribing and register as independent prescribers in their own right.

This builds on the medical background and understanding of medications, which nurses have, and most of the other CAMHS professions (psychologists, psychotherapists, social workers and AHPs) do not, making nurses a natural avenue for enhancing the capacity of the service, particularly in areas like ADHD clinics, which can be very labour intensive, given the need for regular reviews of medication and physical health monitoring. There remains a debate within nursing as to whether this element of expanded role is actually an expansion of nursing, or an encroachment into the medical realm of prescribing. Historically, this debate has focused on whether this effectively makes advanced nurse practitioners into 'mini-doctors', performing a prescribing and monitoring role on a more cost-effective basis, or whether they were actually 'maxi-nurses', allowed more autonomy and using the prescribing function as an adjunct to a more central nursing focus (Castledine 1995).

If one of medical consultant's claims to exclusivity in their role has been eroded with the widespread implementation of independent prescribing by nursing and other professions, then the introduction of the role of Responsible Clinician to replace the medically exclusive Responsible Medical Officer, as part of the 2007 review of the MHA has also opened up the opportunity for CAMHS nurses to take over that role, and higher level of responsibility. So far, this has occurred in very limited places, and needs to be evaluated as to effectiveness and effect on the nurses involved, but it is an exciting development in terms of role expansion.

1.9 CYP_IAPT and the Current Genericization of Roles

Elsewhere in this book we will see in more detail how roles in community CAMHS have changed over the last few years in England through the introduction of the programme of Children and Young People's Increasing Access to Psychological Therapies (CYP_IAPT). Whilst I am about to make some very specific criticisms of this programme and its effect on nursing in particular, I need to stress that CYP-IAPT has been an overwhelmingly positive programme for CAMHS in England. Based, in part, on the adult mental health programme of Increasing Access to Psychological Therapies (IAPT), it has dramatically changed the level of funding available to CAMHS by demonstrating an increased adherence to evidence-based therapeutic approaches, and using this as a lever to increase funding. Led by the Anna Freud Centre, the initial CAMHS Outcome Research Consortia (CORC) introduced the use of Routine Outcome Measures (ROMs) as a way of demonstrating effectiveness of treatment for children and young people, and gave evidence of the utility of therapies within our population, laying the groundwork for a roll-out of the wider CYP_IAPT programme across England. In many ways, this standardised approach to therapeutic intervention, and crucially a centralised collection of data, has put CAMHS ahead of adult mental health in the UK, and provides a much better standardised provision of evidence-based care pathways than is available elsewhere. Within the programme nurses have been seen as ideal candidates for the advanced training in CBT and systemic therapies, which primarily contribute to those pathways, because of their existing skillset. Other professional groups have also undertaken CYP_IAPT training too, and emphasized conformity to the model, as is always the case in evidence-based models of care. What it has also arguably done, however, is to further erode the distinctive ways in which nurses enact different therapies, and emphasized instead the importance of generic skills. Whilst this programme has been very clear that it is different from the somewhat manualized version of CBT, which is the practice in the adult version of IAPT, it has also ensured that levels of training offered are those deemed necessary to the task, rather than allowing nurses and others to train to Masters level proficiency and full registration as psychotherapists.

1.10 Summary

This chapter has looked at the way CAMH nursing has developed, mainly out of a broader tradition of mental health nursing, as a way of understanding underlying conceptual frameworks and their contribution to the use of nursing skills within child and adolescent mental health. The principle themes we have examined are those of relationship-building, 'caring', 'ordinariness', an holistic approach, and knowledge of the medical model of psychiatry. There is a recognition that the overlap of skills and approaches that occurs in mental health teams, and particularly in

CAMHS is much more than in physical healthcare teams. This is particularly important in the 'generic' element of CAMHS work, which constitutes a higher proportion of the overall task. There is also some understanding that the individual personalities and other personal qualities of the people who take on nursing and other roles in some ways shape their approach to the work. Although there are hints of commonality with other mental health professions and with the wider professional groupings, there is a clear lack of definition of whether nurses do anything different to the other professions, or whether *they perform a similar task, but in a different and distinctive way*. The policy context, we have seen, has a push towards a generic focus on skills and competencies, rather than the traditional multidisciplinary construction of teams, and it remains important for nurses to be able to verbalise what they do and to be able to value the contribution they have to distressed young people though the distinctive approach that they bring to the function of CAMHS. Throughout the rest of the book, we will return to the core theme of how these apparently simple nursing skills bring an indispensable value to young people's experience.

> **Box 1.1 What Are Nursing Strengths?**
> - Mental health nursing and CAMH nursing share some of wider nursing's focus on physical healthcare, and knowledge of the medical systems, medications and model of care.
> - Peplau and others focused on the therapeutic relationship and 'therapeutic use of self' as a way of engaging and working with people, and most nurses use this as a primary focus of their way of working with people.
> - Nurses provide 24/7 care in a way that other professions do not, so the effect of 'being there' for the whole journey gives a different perspective on how actively nurses need to engage. This also explains a focus on 'therapeutic milieu', creating conditions for change.
> - Nursing tends not to take an expert position, and will work 'alongside' people rather than doing things *to* them, so non-directive approaches come naturally to most nurses. Nurses' 'ordinariness' and caring focus positions them differently in relation to children and young people.
> - This allows an advocacy position to be taken by nurses, which enables people to take up new approaches to thinking and access services that they may have struggled to do alone.

References

Adams D (1982) Life the universe, and everything. Pan Books, London
Allan HT (2002) Nursing the clinic, being there and hovering: ways of caring in a British fertility clinic. J Adv Nurs 38(1):86–93
Appleton C (1993) The art of nursing: the experience of nurses and patients. J Adv Nurs 18:892–899

Baldwin L (2002) The nursing role in out-patient child and adolescent mental health services. J Clin Nurs 11:520–525

Baldwin L (2005) Multi-disciplinary post-registered education in child and adolescent mental health services. Nurse Educ Today 25:17–22

Baldwin L (2008) The discourse of professional identity in child and adolescent mental health services. University of Nottingham, E-theses. http://eprints.nottingham.ac.uk/10504/. Accessed 19 Apr 2019

Barker P, Reynolds W, Ward T (1995) The proper focus of nursing: a critique of the "caring" ideology. Int J Nurs Stud 32(4):386–397

Barker P, Jackson S, Stevenson C (1999) The need for psychiatric nursing: towards a multidimensional theory of caring. Nurs Inq 6:103–111

Bhoyrub JB, Morton HG (1983) Psychiatric problems in childhood. A guide for nurses. Pitman, London

BMJ (2016) A career in child and adolescent psychiatry. https://www.bmj.com/content/354/bmj. i4983. Accessed 19 Apr 2019

Case M (2019) How to treat people: a nurse at work. Viking/Penguin Books, London

Castledine G (1995) Will the nurse practitioner be a mini doctor or a maxi nurse? Br J Nurs 4(16):938–939

Crawford P, Nolan P, Brown B (1998) Ministering to madness: the narratives of people who have left religious orders to work in the caring professions. J Adv Nurs 28(1):212–220

Croom S (2001) Making a difference to child and adolescent mental health: the nursing contribution. Department of Health, London. (Unpublished)

Davies J, Cresswell A, Hannigan B (2002) Child and adolescent mental health services: rhetoric and reality. Paediatr Nurs 14(3):26–28

Delaney K (1992) Nursing in child psychiatric milieus: part 1. What nurses do. J Child Adolesc Psychiatr Ment Health Nurs 5(1):10–14

DH (1994) Working in partnership: a collaborative approach to care. Department of Health, London

DH (2004) National Service Framework for children, young people and maternity services: change for children-every child matters. Department of Health/Department for Education and Skills, London

DH (2005) Chief Nursing Officer's review of mental health nursing: consultation document. Department of Health, London

DH (2006) From values to action: the Chief Nursing Officer's review of mental health nursing. Department of Health, London

Dhogra N, Parkin A, Frake C, Gale F (2001) A multidisciplinary handbook of child and adolescent mental health for front-line professionals. Jessica Kingsley Publishers Ltd., London

Duffy D, Lee R (1998) Mental health nursing today: ideal and reality. Ment Health Pract 1(8):14–16

Faulconbridge J, Hunt K, Laffan A (2018) Improving the psychological wellbeing of children and young people: effective prevention and early intervention across health, education and social care. Jessica Kingsley Publishers, London

FitzGibbon S, Holyoake D (2002) Discussing child and adolescent mental health nursing. APS Publishing, Salisbury

Geanellos R (1999) The milieu and milieu therapy in adolescent mental health nursing. Int J Psychiatr Nurs Res 5(3):638–648

Gilbert P (2005) Compassion: conceptualisations, research and use in psychotherapy. Routledge, London

Gournay K (1995) What to do with nursing models. J Psychiatr Ment Health Nurs 2:325–327

Graham IW (2001) Seeking a clarification of meaning: a phenomenological interpretation of the craft of mental health nursing. J Psychiatr Ment Health Nurs 8:335–345

Haldane JD (1963) The functions, selection and training of the nurse in a residential psychiatric unit for children. J Nurs Stud 1:27–36

Haldane JD, Lindsay SF, Smith JD (1971) Nursing in child, adolescent and family psychiatry. Int J Nurs Stud 8:91–102

Hogarth C (1991) Adolescent psychiatric nursing. Mosby Year Book, St. Louis

Horrocks P (1986) Bridges over troubled waters: a report from the NHS Advisory Service on Services for Disturbed Adolescents. The NHS Health Advisory Service, London

Lacey I (1999) The role of the child primary mental health worker. J Adv Nurs 30(1):220–228

Leddy S, Pepper JM (1993) Conceptual bases of nursing, 3rd edn. J.B. Lippincott, Philadelphia

Leighton S, Smith C, Minns K, Crawford P (2001) Specialist child and adolescent: a force to be reckoned with? Ment Health Pract 5(2):8–13

Limerick M, Baldwin L (2000) Nursing in outpatient child and adolescent mental health. Nurs Stand 15(13–15):43–45

McDougall T (2005) Child and adolescent mental health services in the UK: nurse consultants. J Child Adolesc Psychiatr Nurs 18(2):79–83

McDougall T (2006) Child and adolescent mental health nursing. Blackwell, Oxford

McDougall T, Armstrong M, Trainor G (2010) Helping children and young people who self-harm: an introduction to self-harming and suicidal behaviours for health professionals. Routledge, London

McMorrow R (1990) The new clinicians. Sr Nurse 10(3):22–23

Mental Health Foundation (1999) Bright futures: promoting children and young people's mental health. Mental Health Foundation, London

Nightingale F (1859) Notes on nursing: what it is, and what it is not. Harrison, London

Nolan P (1993) A history of mental health nursing. Chapman and Hall, London

Onyett S, Pillinger T, Muijen M (1995) Making community health teams work. The Sainsbury Centre for Mental Health, London

Peplau HE (1982) Interpersonal techniques: the crux of psychiatric nursing. In: Smoyak S, Rouslin S (eds) A collection of classics in psychiatric nursing literature. Charles B. Slack Inc., New Jersey

Pierson J (2011) Understanding social work: history and context. Open University Press, Milton Keynes

Pilgrim D, Rogers A (1994) Service users' views of psychiatric nurses. Br J Nurs 3(1):16–18

Price J, McAlinden O (2017) Essentials of nursing children and young people. Sage Publications, London

Puskar K, Lamb J, Martsolf DS (1990) The role of the psychiatric/mental health nurse clinical specialist in an Adolescent Coping Skills Group. J Child Adolesc Psychiatr Nurs 3(2): 47–51

RCOT (2019) What is occupational therapy? Royal College of Occupational Therapists. https://www.rcot.co.uk/about-occupational-therapy/what-is-occupational-therapy. Accessed 19 Apr 2019

Repper J (2000) Adjusting the focus of mental health nursing: incorporating service users' experience of recovery. J Ment Health 9(6):575–587

Rutter M (1986) Child psychiatry: looking 30 years ahead. Child Psychol Psychiatry 27(6):803–841

Ryan N, McDougall T (2008) Nursing children and young people with ADHD. Routledge, London

Sainsbury Centre (1997) Pulling together: the future roles and training of mental health staff. The Sainsbury Centre for Mental Health, London

Sainsbury Centre (2001) The capable practitioner. The Sainsbury Centre for Mental Health, London

Scharer K (1999) Nurse-parent relationship building in a child psychiatric unit. J Child Adolesc Psychiatr Nurs 12(4):153–167

Stickley T, Spandler H (2014) Compassion and mental health nursing. In: Stickley T, Wright N (eds) Theories for mental health nursing: a guide for practice. Sage Publications, London

Tilley S (1999) Altschul's legacy in mediating British and American psychiatric nursing discourses: common sense and the 'absence' of the accountable practitioner. J Psychiatr Ment Health Nurs 6:283–295

Townley M (2002) Mental health needs of children. Nurs Stand 16(30):38–46

Walker L, Jackson S, Barker P (1998) Perceptions of the psychiatric nurse's role: a pilot study. Nurs Stand 12(16):35–38

Watson J (1985) Nursing: the philosophy and science of caring. University of Colorado Press, Colorado

Wilkinson T (1983) Child and adolescent psychiatric nursing. Blackwell, Oxford

Wright K, McKeown M (2018) Essentials of mental health nursing. Sage Publications, London

Chapter 2
What Do Children and Young People Want and Need from Nurses (and Therapists?)

Leanne Walker

with Danni and Hannah

2.1   Introduction

Within the field of children and young people's mental health, consulting children and young people in what it is that they want and need within their healthcare is a growing area (Royal College of Nursing 2014: 6). In more recent years, it has gained increasing momentum. The field is progressively moving towards collaborative practice with not just children and young people, but also with their families and carers. Perhaps sometimes as adults, we can lose sight of what it is that children and young people want and need in healthcare settings. Often, this is not done on purpose; we just grow older and further away from childhood. At times we can make assumptions based on what we think it is that children and young people want and need. Sometimes, these are correct, sometimes not, and when they are not it is often not due to bad intent. Of course, the only true way of knowing what children and young people want and need from nurses and therapists is to ask them. Those with lived experience often know what went well and what did not go so well in their care and this should be used to invoke change in practice and within services. Additionally, it is important to consult a broad range of children and young people and hold in mind those that are hard or harder to engage, as they can offer valuable insights (Claveirole 2004: 258). Certainly it is essential to remember that what one child or young person might want or need, another might not. Likewise, what works well in one area of the country might not in another (Care Quality Commission 2018a: 5). Cultures, of course, differ.

L. Walker (✉)
Derbyshire Healthcare NHS Foundation Trust, Derbyshire, UK

© Springer Nature Switzerland AG 2020
L. Baldwin (ed.), *Nursing Skills for Children and Young People's Mental Health*,
https://doi.org/10.1007/978-3-030-18679-1_2

2.2 Lived Experience

It goes without saying, within and outside of healthcare, we are all distinct individuals with varying needs (Royal College of Nursing 2003: 2). Although we can look at experiences and collate themes, it is important that we never lose sight of this individuality. This chapter will use lived experience supported by academia, policies and reports to explore what it is that children and young people want and need from nurses and therapists. However, as previously implied, individuality suggests there can never be a 'routine' approach as what works for one person may not work for another (Sellman 2011: 20) and this should be kept in mind throughout. Firstly, I shall look upon my own lived experience within Child and Adolescent Mental Health Services (CAMHS), before moving on to other lived experience. Having accessed CAMHS as a teenager, I have my own opinions around what it is that children and young people want and need from nurses and therapists. Of course, I am just one person and this is only my own singular experience. I had my first appointment at CAMHS at age 15, prior to this, I didn't even know CAMHS existed. I didn't stay in the service long, but shortly was re-referred and then I didn't leave the service as a service user until after my 19th birthday. To put it simply, my first experience of the service was bad (and short lived fortunately) but I didn't know it was poor at the time, as I had nothing to compare it with. I didn't know it was supposed to be, or even could be any different. To me, the worker I saw felt patronising, showed little empathy and I was made to feel as if my problems were minimal in comparison to others. Ultimately, I became disengaged and left feeling unheard and frustrated. During the time period that I accessed CAMHS, I worked with a range of professionals within a range of settings including 1 to 1 and group. At 15, as a young person sat in front of a mental health professional (any professional for that matter), I didn't know what it was that I wanted or needed from these individuals. I took whatever I was given to be what I thought I *needed*. I assumed whatever I was told to be the truth or the right way of doing something, because after all, they were the experts. That is the way I saw it then. It was only after I'd been in the service for a while and seen a few different professionals that I could begin to see what I not only wanted but needed from the people I was working with. It was only in hindsight after leaving the service and reflecting on my experiences as a whole, that I was able to draw out the fundamental elements that I needed in order to move forward and progress within my life.

I doubt that any of the themes in this chapter will come as a surprise. I hope to cement some of the key qualities of nurses and therapists. These can, in an ever-changing environment at CAMHS, be overlooked or overshadowed by other matters. For me, most of what I needed evolved around the individual worker's personality and attitude. Being able to connect with the person I was working with was the single most important factor. In my own experience, genuine connection equalled progress, with no exception. Establishing a good working relationship came alongside other key components—time and space. I needed the worker to give me enough time, in order to build a relationship, to then feel able to share all the difficult things I was struggling with. I shall discuss these components and more, in further detail later on in the chapter. Next are some thoughts from Danni around her own lived experience.

2.3 Reflections from Lived Experience

As my own lived experience comes purely from a community setting, the chapter turns to Danni who brings a different perspective. As a young person, Danni was admitted into an inpatient unit and here she reflects on her own personal experience.

> *In mental healthcare, one of the most significant skills a nurse can possess is to care. As young individuals require nurture and time to explain what is distressing them and guidance that recovery can be an achieved aspiration. As it can be an especially frightening time, being admitted into hospital no matter the distance from a child or young person's home. This is due to being in unfamiliar surroundings, with unfamiliar people who are also poorly and may act or display behaviours that could trigger or distress other young people within that hospital setting. Personalised daily goals supported my recovery, that were encouraged by nursing staff. Each day, I would document an improvement to view that I was slowly moving forward. This supported my recovery as it enabled me to slowly adjust to my situation, instead of frightening myself with a larger picture that did not feel achievable.*
>
> *The balance between being treated as a child or as an adult is extremely important, especially whilst being an adolescent. This is because a young person requires additional support in certain areas, such as maintaining safety, yet requires additional independence. Nursing staff always addressed me with a realistic, but fair attitude. This skill is significantly important to adopt as young individuals commonly act against advice or support due to their age, not just their illness. Maintaining this attitude is important as nurses hold responsibility over their patients care and may in certain situations take away advantages due to a situation that has occurred, yet there needs to be flexibility within this to ensure that these measures have been taken correctly.*
>
> *Utilizing an empathetic approach is paramount within mental health nursing. Children and young people do not always understand the situation in which they are placed and this can cause a high proportion of distress. Communicating with young people on their level and conversing with them in an array of activities that they enjoy, enables a therapeutic relationship with young people to develop. This supports nurses to analyse further into any factors that could be influencing young individuals mental health, such as: family, relationships, finance etc.*

Danni's reflection draws out that accessing mental health services can be a scary time for children and young people. However, for a nurse or a therapist, the setting is their everyday job, so perhaps the awareness of this can be unintentionally lost. Having now had my own experience of working within CAMHS (as an expert by experience) I have found myself understanding how easy it is to lose sight of the smaller things which make a huge difference simply because, as a member of staff, they become routine. Danni also highlights the importance of balance between being treated as a child, adolescent or young adult. Interestingly, it appears the core to Danni's reflection centre around interpersonal skills of the nurse or therapist; being caring, nurturing and empathic.

2.4   What Is It That Children and Young People Want and Need? Key Themes

Although the nursing field is one that has changed and does change over time, it appears certain elements remain the same, such as the need to be caring and having passion for the role (Peate 2012). When it comes to what children and young people want, Collins et al. (2017: 163) found personal attributes are favoured over information and skill sets. If there was a choice, for example, between the qualities of a physical CAMHS building and individuals qualities, from the above experiences already and from my experiences of others, children and young people care less about environmental issues such as room design, and more about things such as 'Can I open up to this person?', 'Is this person nice?', etc.

This chapter now turns to the key themes drawn out from collective experience, my own, experiences of fellow young people who became friends, family, work colleagues, acquaintances, children and young people from a range of mental health settings including inpatient and community. They have been collated into the following headings: Consistency, Being Given Time, Working Relationship, Communication, Interpersonal Skills, Participation, Flexibility and Continuance of Care/Good Transitions. In no order of importance, they shall now be discussed in more depth, using examples to illustrate.

2.5   Consistency

Whether this is in regard to community CAMHS or inpatient, consistency is a very important aspect to children and young people and a lot of the time is highly valued. This usually relates to consistency in terms of having a single named worker, as opposed (or preferably) to say having appointments in the same place, at the same time every week (although some consistency in this way can be important too). Of course, it is inevitable that people are off work from time to time and as a whole this is generally accepted. It is common knowledge that we all get ill or need to take a holiday. It's when children or young people see a different worker time and time again with little or no explanation that it becomes an issue. Perhaps this highlights transparency as important also, in terms of offering a simple explanation if this is to be the case such as 'there is a lot of staff illness at the moment...'. There can be a frustration in not having an explanation.

Having consistency in terms of worker is important to children and young people for a multitude of reasons. Firstly, seeing someone new all of the time, for example for every appointment or every other appointment, often means they have to retell their story time and time again. Of course, this is not only repetitive and somewhat tiresome, but also can be traumatic, such as having to relive bad experiences so the new worker can understand. Secondly, having to explain everything all over again can also sometimes mean little is actually gained from the session, as the bulk of the time is taken up retelling. From my experiences, children and young people want to see someone who really knows who they are, what they have experienced and what they are currently experiencing. Someone who can pick up where they last left off. Perhaps this is because that one person will then have a more in-depth understanding, not just of the child or young person but of their circumstances and the wider impact of happenings within their life. Thirdly, only so much can be gathered from reading a child or young person's notes and sometimes perhaps these notes can lack in the real emotion and feelings of an individual or situation. Of course, if there is no consistency, there is also the matter of opening up to essentially what is a stranger at every appointment, which can be a huge difficulty in itself and not just for child or young person. This point links nicely to 'time' as another key component which shall be discussed following an example from Hannah, a young person who has accessed mental health services.

> Once a young person has created a bond with a worker, it's incredibly important to their support system. Consistency is key. However, it's important to appreciate that they may not 'click' with the first worker they meet. It took me meeting 5 or 6 different psychologists before I found one I was comfortable speaking to. Once I found that person, I felt I could be a lot more open and productive during our sessions. While I appreciate that resources are often limited, allowing a young person flexibility to find the best source of support for them, but to then give them consistency when things are working, should be a key principle of their care.

2.6 Being Given Time

Here, in this context, being given time is being taken to mean a period of getting to know the child or young person that an individual is working with. In some circumstances or for some children or young people, opening up and feeling able to talk to someone they have just met can be easier than talking to someone who they perhaps know better. However, for many children and young people they need time to get to know the person they are working with so they become more than a stranger. For many, it is hard to tell the entirety of life struggles and experiences to a near complete stranger and there are little other circumstances when this is expected in life. For some children and young people, this could mean a few additional sessions to what is seen as expected. For others this could be a bit of time talking about hobbies and free time instead of diving straight into difficulties. For others, learning small pieces of information about the person they are working with can be of benefit. This doesn't have to be personal, it could be about their job role, or time they have worked in the service for Hannah puts it like this:

> For me personally, being given time was crucial and in reality I needed months of this. After being in the service for a few weeks, discharge was being spoken about. It wasn't that I was ready to leave the service, it was that I hadn't felt able to speak about things that had felt difficult yet. I'd had a change in worker and hadn't been able to reach a place where I was

to feel comfortable in talking. It wasn't until I was given a bit more time, that I was able to trust the person I was working with and then felt able to speak more openly. Time for me was the difference between leaving the service without treatment and having treatment which changed my life completely.

The themes discussed so far, consistency and time, go hand in hand with the third to be discussed here, developing a working relationship.

2.7 Working Relationship

It can be argued that without a good working relationship with the child or young person, little therapeutic work can take place (Ungar et al. 2017: 278). It can be hoped that with consistency and time, a working relationship would develop but that is not necessarily always the case. Other components have been found to be of importance such as the notion of 'mentalisation' (Fuggle et al. 2013: 109). Sometimes a relationship comes naturally, just as some people in life we instantly get on with, but sometimes a therapeutic relationship requires a little more work. As previously stated, in my own experiences establishing a good working relationship was of upmost importance. Although it is assumed that anyone within the nursing or therapeutic profession can be trusted, it sometimes can be an area of difficulty for example, conflicting wants and needs such as that of confidentiality and when it needs to be breached (Sellman 2011: 18). This in turn can impact the working relationship. Children and young people need clarity of what kinds of information will need to be passed onto who. If information has to be passed on to a safeguarding team and the child or young person does not want it to and was not aware such information had to be, this can lead to feelings of mistrust (Sellman 2011: 18). Children and young people need nurses and therapists to take time to establish a good working relationship with foundations of trust which includes a level of honesty and/or transparency. Lastly, here is a reflection from Danni following her experiences within an inpatient unit.

> *Young people require good working relationships with nurses as the comforts that they are accustomed to (home, family, friends, belongings) are taken away and are set upon in a routined approach to aid their recovery. This approach however can prevent or slow down recovery. Young people need these relationships to support them with their wider needs as well as therapy for their mental well-being. They require support in wider aspects of well-being, such as maintaining their safety as they are vulnerable due to their illness. They also require support to live a healthy lifestyle, possess healthy relationships and develop living skills such as cooking and budgeting to enhance independence and recovery and reduce the risk of relapse.*

Danni highlights the importance of good working relationships with nurses in an inpatient setting, especially given that other kinds of relationship often are across distance. Danni also highlights different areas of life that young people need support with, perhaps good working relationships would also depend upon communication between different workers and services supporting within these areas.

2.8 Communication

In this section, communication will be taken to mean how information is shared by the nurse or therapist with other people, services or organisations working with the child or young person. What information is shared, where and with who; who know what. When consulting service users, families and carers in what it is that they want from nurses, good communication has been a highlighted area (Rush and Cook 2013). Time and time again, I've heard the phrase 'wish they (staff and services) communicated better'. Again, as the previous section highlighted, this suggests nurses and therapists need to have a degree of transparency in the work they do. As a service user, I knew extremely little about what went on 'behind the scenes' such as discussions in supervision or team meetings. In reality, I had little idea who knew what.

Communication is especially important when there is more than one team or organisation working with the child, young people or family. Joint working can be of benefit in some cases, for example CAMHS and social care. Good communication between different teams is vital as the example below highlights.

> During my time within CAMHS, I also had a range of other professionals who were working with me from outside of CAMHS. On occasion there were meetings where everyone working with me were invited together. Therefore, I assumed that everyone told everyone everything. That is to say, that communication was in a loop. For example, if I told my CAMHS worker something then they would tell the other professionals and vice versa. It was only after leaving the service that I discovered that this was not the case. It is important that what is shared with who is very clear to the child or young person. As for me, I rarely repeated myself to other professionals if I had said something once to one, as I really thought it was shared with the others and didn't know otherwise. This could have been rectified with a few sentences of explanation or a conversation from one of my workers explaining what information is shared and what is not.

2.9 Interpersonal Skills

Interpersonal skills should not be seen as less important than other competing aspects within care. Perhaps having good interpersonal skills is the foundation to what children and young people want and need. Sergeant (Sergeant 2009: 47) came up with a whole list of interpersonal skills that are valued by children and young people: 'trust, commitment, unconditional positive regard, genuineness, honesty, support, responsiveness, consistency, confidentiality, non-judgemental attitude'. Of course, it is one thing knowing these but another putting them into practice. For example, there is a fine line between confidentiality and trust but perhaps that is where other skills come in such as having a level of honesty with the child or young person. For example, a nurse tells a 14-year-old that they can trust them. This prompts the young person to tell the nurse they have been dating someone who is 17 years old. The nurse has to tell the parent to make sure the young person is kept safe so calls them in but doesn't explain any of this to the young person. The young person shuts down and then does not tell the therapist anymore. The trust is broken. The outcome may have been different if the nurse had an open conversation about what kinds of information needs to be shared and why it needs to be shared, including how any information is shared if it needs to be. For example, the young person could share it with their parent, the nurse could share it or they could share it together. It can take a lot of courage for a young person to speak about things in their life and it can be extremely discouraging to have finally done this and then the outcome is felt as negative for the young person. It is important that the young person can make an informed decision before sharing the information, so the working relationship remains intact.

An absolute key skill which has yet to be discussed is empathy and mastering correct levels. In a good working relationship, empathy is vital (Fuggle et al. 2013: 108). There is a balance which will vary depending on each individual person that work is being engaged with. Deploying this skill correctly has been found to be linked to overall outcomes, in particular, clinicians having lower empathy to less change and higher disengagement rates (Moyers and Miller 2013: 878). Services can fall into seeing children, young people and families as numbers such as numbers on waiting lists or when reporting statistics such as number of sessions received, numbers of 'did not attend' or 'was not brought'. How empathy and emotion are used is important. For example, a child shares that another child has been picking on them and how upset it made them, the therapist asks them if they told a teacher and they say no. Conversation moves on. How the upset is reflected back is key, not being void of emotion and knowing as a nurse or therapist you have feelings too. In some situations, it can be of benefit to share small parts of personal experiences. For me, this always validated my feelings and made me feel like I wasn't the only one experiencing what I was. It also gave me hope that things had changed for the person I was sat with, so they could for me. Of course there is a line in which someone can overshare and I guess that is the skill part.

2.10   Participation

Participation within the CAMHS field is usually taken to mean the involvement of children, young people and their parents and carers. This could be involvement within their care or within the service. It includes service improvement and development and generally anything else to do with the service. For example, choosing what time of day suits best for their appointments, opportunities to say when things are not going so well and being taken seriously when they are not. Or this could mean more broadly, such as having a voice in how the service operates, for example by having opportunities to sit on interview panels to ensure the right people are employed for the service. This goes all the way to how services are commissioned (Williams et al. 2017). For this to not be tokenistic, there must be an overall structure in place and a real readiness to make these changes (Worrall-Davies 2008). In my experience, opportunities to be involved were of near equal importance to the interventions I was receiving, especially towards the end of treatment. Children and young people need nurses and therapists to allow them to actively participate such as helping to make decisions within their own care (Royal College of Nursing 2003). This of course means that nurses and therapists within young people's mental health services need to be given the tools, time and or relevant training in order to facilitate this (Royal College of Nursing 2014: 8). In her own words, Hannah explains what participation gave to her.

> *The power of participation in both an individual's care and in the wider improvement of a service is vital. For me, having a say in my own treatment made me feel more motivated to engage with the support I was being offered and therefore made it much more successful. Even with small things, such as an activity we could do while we talked or even setting my goals in collaboration with my team. I also found that participating in wider service improvement gave me a sense of purpose when I needed one most. It gave me much of the confidence back that being ill had caused me to lose and I felt like I was achieving things and that I was worth something. It's a huge misconception that young people don't care, or don't want to have a say. But by just asking little questions and encouraging an open dialogue between the service user and their treatment team, care can be a lot more personal and efficient.*

Hannah's example highlights what a difference active involvement can have, not just in a child or young person's care but more broadly in their life. On a personal perspective, participation changed my life completely. It opened up many doors and opportunities for me and gave me the tools to reach out and take those chances. Firstly, I was supported to attend a participation group, where fellow service users and staff met to discuss ways to improve the service. Here I developed confidence, social skills, but most importantly, I met the people who were to become my close friends. This is a massive, lifelong impact that I have gained from the service. Ultimately, within my care, participation showed me that my voice mattered and like Hannah, that I was worth something. This was huge and enabled me to go forward with my life.

2.11 Flexibility

Here flexibility is being taken to mean a few things. Firstly, in terms of being seen in a service at the right time. Sometimes as a nurse or therapist it is important to recognise when it might not be the right time for a child or young person to engage in work together. For example because a child or young person has made it to the top of the waiting list, doesn't necessarily mean they are at a place to receive treatment. Sometimes environments outside of therapy make it difficult for therapeutic work to be achieved together. Sometimes therapy doesn't seem to be progressing in a way it is thought it could and sometimes the child or young person doesn't engage no matter what techniques have been tried. At these times children and young people need to know that it is okay to postpone therapy or work until a later date. Acknowledging that this is okay can be of importance due to pressures of often having waited so long on a waiting list, so feeling as if the service has to be accepted while it is being offered.

Secondly, in terms of right place, this could be in relation to appointment time or location. Regardless of service constraints such as how many children or young people there are to be seen, flexibility is of importance. It has been found that sometimes having appointments in a clinic can prevent attendance (Department of Health 2015: 44). Young people can sometimes find it hard to physically travel to buildings, sometimes there is significant worry about going to a new place, within a new setting and meeting new people for the first time and this is without the lingering stigma regarding attending mental health clinics. Children and young people want nurses and therapists to recognise this and where possible, have some flexibility in supporting appointment attendance. Going to a person's home or meeting elsewhere such as in school can be of benefit. Again, not one same approach works for everyone. Thirdly, some children and young people want family, parents or carers involved and others do not. Often it can be assumed that families or carers should automatically be involved but for some, involvement can be counterproductive. It is very important not to assume involvement and have careful discussions around this with the young person. The level of involvement should also not be assumed to be static but fluid meaning that it could change over time. Finally, flexibility could be in terms of being able to admit when things are not going well with the individual worker and being able to work with someone else instead. However, Hannah captures the difficulties surrounding this.

> The ability to be flexible comes from having a good dialogue between the service user and their care team and perhaps also with their family. They [child or young person] need to feel comfortable enough to admit they don't feel they can be open with someone and would like to try to speak with someone else. It kind of goes with the things about interpersonal skills. Unless a young person feels comfortable saying they don't 'click' with a worker, then there's no point having the flexibility. Obviously it's a really individual thing. Point I'm trying to make is that consistency in having the same worker is important, but the wrong kind of consistency (i.e. with a care team you can't engage with) is detrimental.

Hannah highlights the way different wants and needs interlink. Children and young people want flexibility in worker in order to find the person which works for them. However, if the worker is unable to recognise when things are not going as planned, perhaps having flexibility in this regard is pointless. This shows again the importance of interpersonal skills and being acutely aware of them.

2.12 Continuance of Care/Good Transitions

Here, transition is being taken to mean the move from CAMHS to adult services. Not all children and young people go on to need a service after young people's services, but for those who do, in my experiences transition can be a difficult time and continuation of care is important to young people and their families. In recent years, it has been recognised that transition from young peoples to adult services is currently poor overall (Paul et al. 2015: 437). Time and time again young people have been found to have been failed at this time (House of Commons 2018: 15). Of course, it goes without saying that birthdays can be predicted and as most CAMHS have an upper age limit (House of Commons 2018: 15), when young people need to transition should not come as a surprise. All too often I have heard stories of transition not being considered until right at the last minute and then it is rushed and not thought through. I have also heard young people not being involved in the process or being told things such as they won't meet the threshold for adult services anyway. Even worse, being told they still need support but just discharged and told if there are any problems to go back to their general practice. I have found that often young people are left feeling alone and unsure of where to turn. 'Adolescent transition Care' (Royal College of Nursing 2013) reported similar findings. Danni's example below brings a different perspective of transition which is of equal importance, the role nurses play transitioning young people from inpatient services to outpatient.

> The role nurses should play transitioning young people into outpatient treatment is hugely correlated into communication and the expectations of support that should be carried into outpatient support. My experience highlighted the lack of communication between multidisciplinary teams in supporting a child or adolescent once discharged. This is a serious issue that needs to be addressed as it can be a very traumatising experience being discharged into community care and can have serious/fatal consequences. Nurses should also address relapse prevention support with young people, before they get discharged into the community. As I never received this and believe that this is a significant tool to reduce the likelihood of relapsing.

As Danni's example alludes to, leaving a service, just like coming into a service for the first time, can be difficult for some children and young people. Acknowledging this and doing what work is possible to minimise this is perhaps of importance.

2.13 What Do Policies and Reports Say?

The majority of what has been reflected upon so far has focused mainly around lived experiences. Lived experience rightly so often finds itself within reports, policies and academia and this is where the chapter now turns, in order to further explore the wants and needs of children and young people of nurses and therapists. There are an abundance of reports and publications that state or suggest that children and young people need care which puts the person at the centre (Royal College of Nursing 2003, Department of Health 2015, Care Quality Commission 2018a). The National Health Service Regulations themselves (National Health Service, England 2013) stipulate patients should be at the 'heart' of services. Future in Mind (Department of Health 2015: 11) set out clearly that children and young people are experts in their own care and that services should offer opportunities for children and young people to regularly assess whether treatment is going well or not and make changes accordingly. It has been found that better care can be provided when children and young person are actively involved within decisions (Care Quality Commission 2018a: 9) and perhaps active involvement cannot be achieved without being put at the centre of care. If a child or young person is put at the centre of care, aspects of participation and collaborative working should come naturally. For example, a nurse referred 'Tamara' to a weekly group therapy session. 'Tamara' decided not to go, not because she didn't want support but she wasn't really sure what the sessions were, who would be there and she'd never been to the building it was in before. 'Tamara' was not put at the centre of care and subsequently her voice not heard. The nurse recorded it as 'Did Not Attend'. In another scenario, the nurse spoke to 'Tamara' about the group and 'Tamara' decided she would like to give it a try. Together they discussed what it would be like and then her nurse supported her in attending the first session. The decision wasn't made for 'Tamara', she was placed at the centre of her care and her voice was heard showcasing collaborative practice. The Care Quality Commission (2018a) report suggests better care can be provided when this happens, indicating that this is not just of benefit on an individual level but on a whole service level.

When a child or young person is at the centre of care, in theory nothing would happen within their care without influence or communication with the child or young person (and parent or carer if appropriate). If this is unpacked further, it can be related to all the above paragraphs. To illustrate, children or young people would clearly know who knows what, they would be given more time to form a therapeutic relationship if that was needed, transition would be thought about together and started within enough time. What a child wanted and needed in each individual circumstance, across all aspects and levels of care, would be considered. Like most things however, there is a line here. For example, a young person in cognitive behavioural therapy doesn't want to do any homework or exposure, a therapist agrees seeing it as putting the young person at the centre of care but this leads to minimal learning and defeats the object of the therapy (Fuggle et al. 2013: 116). Continuously however, participation and active involvement within services is highlighted within policy (Collins et al. 2017: 159). Of course, if it was as simple of putting the child at the centre and this solved everything, CAMHS would already be operating perfectly in this way. However, 'things' get in the way of ideal, sometimes regardless of intent. For example, although the recent report by the Care Quality Commission (2018a: 4) found passionate staff within children and young people's mental health services, they found the system as a whole produced support that is disjointed. Even if the individual worker has the passion and intent to place the child or young person at the centre of care, systems and differences can interfere with that ability. Therefore, even with all the will in the world, nurses and therapists would still struggle to meet what it is that children and young people want and need. The point this highlights is, perhaps the focus should be less on improving/looking at what children and young people want from individual nurses and therapists, and instead looking at the system as a whole and how it fits (or doesn't fit) together in order to achieve this.

Leading from this point, increasingly children and young people need nurses and therapists with creative abilities and solutions to such issues in order to tackle disjointed care and other barriers within and across services as suggested by the Care Quality Commission report (2018a: 5). Creative abilities has not been discussed so far and perhaps isn't something automatically thought about when considering what it is that children and young people want and need from nurses and therapists. Fuggle et al. (2013: 116) outline how creative abilities can also be useful within therapy, such as using role-play and visual communication methods. One area which could be seen as in need of a creative solution is transition from CAMHS. The House of Commons (2018) report suggests children and young people want transitions from CAMHS to adult services to be more joined up. Danni highlighted earlier that transitions between services are also of importance such as that from inpatient to community. The House of Commons (2018: 30) publication found the different systems between services often mean data such as clinical notes are not easily shared. For example, the worker wants the notes to be shared easily but the systems do not allow for this. How this is then managed and ensured perhaps requires some outside of the box thinking. In this example, if it is just taken that the notes can't be shared so that is that, this perhaps leads to things that children and young people don't want such as having to retell their story again and as previously discussed, this is not always a positive experience. Future in Mind (Department of Health 2015: 11) sets out this vision that children and young people should not have to keep repeating their story to different people.

There are a range of publications that have addressed transition between services as an issue. Starting transitions in enough time was highlighted in the publication 'No Health Without Mental Health…' (Department of Health 2011: 25) as important and has been highlighted time and time again since (Department of Health 2014; NICE 2016; Care Quality Commission 2018b). In order to get transition right for each individual child, young person or family, nurses, therapists and mental health workers need to consult with them in enough time and encourage feedback about their experiences following transition. 'Transition from children's to adults' service for young people using health or social care services' is just one guideline which supports this notion (NICE 2016). Adult services are not needed (or even wanted) by some young people and knowing what services are out there as alternatives including how to access them is important. 'Children and young people's mental health—every nurse's business' suggests to begin with *'clear referral pathways are vital'* (Royal College of Nursing 2014: 7). This is to ensure support can be easily accessed when it is needed or services can refer people on to support that is more suitable. For example, after waiting for a year on a waiting list, a family may feel compelled to accept the support even if it is now the wrong time for them. If they knew the support will be there for them, the exact time they needed it, they may feel better about turning down the support at that particular time. The Joint Commissioning Panel for Mental Health (2013: 11) suggests a good CAMHS service would include nurses and therapists signposting children and young people to other services if required. This in turn implies that nurses and therapists should be equipped with local knowledge in order to do this if necessary. Of course ideally, there would not be waiting lists allowing children or young people to access support at the right time without worrying about how long they will be waiting (Joint Commissioning Panel for Mental Health 2013: 11). There is something to be said about how this worry ties in to discharge from services. Perhaps if there was an easy way in, the way out would be more manageable.

One thing is for sure, there will always be a need for services to be different and have different ways of going about things. There will always be a range of people working within a range of services with their own ways of doing things. There will always be people with different ideas, methods and interests but when the wants and needs of the child or young person are put above all of these competing aspects, it becomes easier for nurses, therapists and other workers to care in a way that is joined up, enabling the interests of the child or young person to be at the heart (Care Quality Commission 2018a: 5).

2.14   Summary

When thinking about what it is that is wanted and needed by children and young people from nurses and therapists, it is hard to get away from also talking about services. In some ways, they could be seen as one and the same but in others they differ. It is not the service which has interpersonal skills, or good communication, but the individual staff within the service. Perhaps this chapter has highlighted the importance of service structures in cultivating practices. For example, if there are no procedures in place for active participation and service user feedback, then perhaps individual staff would struggle to do this in a meaningful way. That is to say, a nurse or therapist can be excellent but if the service as a whole is terrible it will leave the care experience not as good as it should or could be. There are a range of components that children and young people both want and need and the use of lived experience throughout this chapter has highlighted that many of these stem from intrinsic qualities of individual nurses and therapists as opposed to environments.

This leaves, for me, the lingering question, are you born a nurse (or therapist), or can you learn to be one? (Peate 2012: 579). However this question is answered, what is important to children and young people is that they (and their families or carers) get the care they need, when they need it, in a way they can access it. That's the important thing for somebody going into this profession, having the drive and passion to want to provide that.

References

Care Quality Commission (2018a) Are we listening? Review of children and young people's mental health services. https://www.cqc.org.uk/sites/default/files/20180308b_arewelistening_report.pdf. Accessed 18 Apr 2019

Care Quality Commission (2018b) BRIEF GUIDE: Transitions out of children and young people's mental health services CQUIN. https://www.cqc.org.uk/sites/default/files/20180228_9001400%20_briefguide-transition_CQUIN.pdf. Accessed 18 Apr 2019

Claveirole A (2004) Listening to young voices: challenges of research with adolescent mental health service users. J Psychiatr Ment Health Nurs 11(3):253–260

Collins R, Notley C, Clarke T, Wilson J, Fowler D (2017) Participation in developing youth mental health services: "Cinderella service" to service re-design. J Public Ment Health 16(4):159–168

Department of Health (2011) No health without mental health: a cross-government mental health outcomes strategy for people of all ages. https://assets.publishing.service.gov.uk/government/uploads/system/uploads/attachment_data/file/213761/dh_124058.pdf. Accessed 18 Apr 2019

Department of Health (2014) Closing the gap: priorities for essential change in mental health. https://assets.publishing.service.gov.uk/government/uploads/system/uploads/attachment_data/file/281250/Closing_the_gap_V2_-_17_Feb_2014.pdf. Accessed 18 Apr 2019

Department of Health (2015) Future in mind. https://assets.publishing.service.gov.uk/government/uploads/system/uploads/attachment_data/file/414024/Childrens_Mental_Health.pdf. Accessed 18 Apr 2019

Fuggle P, Dunsmuir S, Curry V (2013) CBT with children, young people & families. SAGE, London

House of Commons, Education and Health and Social Care Committees (2018) The government's green paper on mental health: failing a generation. https://publications.parliament.uk/pa/cm201719/cmselect/cmhealth/642/642.pdf. Accessed 18 Apr 2019

Joint Commissioning Panel for Mental Health (2013) Guidance for commissioners for child and adolescent mental health services. https://www.jcpmh.info/wp-content/uploads/jcpmh-camhs-guide.pdf. Accessed 18 Apr 2019

Moyers T, Miller W (2013) Is low therapist empathy toxic? Psychol Addict Behav 27(3):878–884

National Health Service, England (2013) The National Health Service (revision of NHS constitution— principles) regulations 2013. http://www.legislation.gov.uk/uksi/2013/317/pdfs/uksi_20130317_en.pdf. Accessed 18 Apr 2019

NICE (2016) Transition from children's to adults' services for young people using health or social care services. https://www.nice.org.uk/guidance/ng43. Accessed 18 Apr 2019

Paul M, Street C, Wheeler N, Singh S (2015) Transition to adult services for young people with mental health needs: a systematic review. Clin Child Psychol Psychiatry 20(3):436–457

Peate I (2012) What makes a good nurse? Br J Nurs 21(10):579–579

Royal College of Nursing (2003) Children and young people's nursing: a philosophy of care, guidance for nursing staff. https://www.rcn.org.uk/-/media/royal-college-of-nursing/documents/publications/2007/october/pub-002012.pdf. Accessed 18 Apr 2019

Royal College of Nursing (2013) Adolescent transition care RCN guidance for nursing staff. 2nd edn. https://www.rcn.org.uk/professional-development/publications/pub-004510. Accessed 18 Apr 2019

Royal College of Nursing (2014) Children and young people's mental health-every nurse's business. https://matrix.rcn.org.uk/__data/assets/pdf_file/0005/587615/004_587_WEB.pdf. Accessed 18 Apr 2019

Rush B, Cook J (2013) What makes a good nurse? Views of patients and carers. Br J Nurs 15(7):382–385

Sellman D (2011) What makes a good nurse: why the virtues are important for nurses. Jessica Kingsley Publishers, London and Philadelphia

Sergeant A (2009) Working within child and adolescent mental health inpatient services. https://www.foundationpsa.org.uk/cms/upload_area/documents/Workingwithinchild andadolescentmentalhealthinpatientservices.pdf. Accessed 18 Apr 2019

Ungar M, Hadfield K, Ikeda J (2017) Adolescents' experiences of therapeutic relationships at high and low levels of risk and resilience. J Soc Work Pract 32(3):277–292

Williams E, Scarisbrick J, Samata B (2017) Increasing participation and involvement. In: McDougall T (ed) Children and young people's mental health essentials for nurses and other professionals. Routledge, Oxon and New York

Worrall-Davies A (2008) Barriers and facilitators to children's and young people's views affecting CAMHS planning and delivery. Child Adolescent Mental Health 13(1):16–18

Chapter 3
Cognitive and Emotional Development of Young People and the Development of Resilience

Laurence Baldwin

3.1 Introduction

We have stressed the need (in Chap. 1) to be aware of the developmental stage of children and young people as a way of informing how we interact with them. This chapter serves as a brief introduction to the complex theories of child and adolescent development and will try and highlight the key points for informing nursing practice. It is necessarily brief, but will give pointers to more in-depth texts and sources of information for follow-up study, and tries to provide a steer for key concepts in a potentially difficult area. In order to do this we need to look both at classic theories of both physical and cognitive development, but also some other concepts that inform certain areas of engaging young people. Identity formation, for example, is a crucial stage of adolescent development which impacts on mental health, so it merits a section of its own, alongside some of the newer thinking about how resilience develops and is potentially very different and individualized. We will also touch on the recent understandings of how early trauma impacts on development and mental health, particularly the concept of 'Adverse Childhood Events' (ACEs).

3.2 Physical Development

Arguably the historic debate about 'nature vs. nurture' starts very early in our lives. Whilst the genetic inheritance we each get from our parents sets a very strong basis for each of us, determining our eye colour, skin tone and physical build, predisposition towards certain conditions, and the conditions in which each foetus develops in the womb also has a bearing on development. When assessing children and young

L. Baldwin (✉)
School of Nursing, Midwifery and Health, Coventry University, Coventry, Warwickshire, UK
e-mail: ac1273@coventry.ac.uk

© Springer Nature Switzerland AG 2020
L. Baldwin (ed.), *Nursing Skills for Children and Young People's Mental Health*,
https://doi.org/10.1007/978-3-030-18679-1_3

people, it is normal to get a developmental history at some point in order to rule out purely physical or organic reasons for what may present as mental health conditions. Pre-birth experiences can shape development in critical ways, so whilst genetics do provide the basic building blocks, what happens to each child's mother during pregnancy can also affect outcomes (Mercer 2018). Although malnutrition is uncommon in the UK, poor diet can have an effect on healthy development. We know that smoking during pregnancy can affect development as well, and excessive intake of alcohol can lead to major difficulties such as Foetal Alcohol Syndrome (FAS). For younger children parents are often quite familiar with recounting the story of their child's early and pre-term existence, and will be expecting some questions on this matter, though some parents do seem to be quite 'unreliable narrators' of their children's early history, due to poor memory or other factors. For young people this line of questioning may seem quite strange, however, and they may not see the relevance of this, in which case it would be best to follow their lead, discuss the current problems, but make a note to return to check any developmental history later, when a therapeutic relationship has been better established and the rationale can be explained. When assessing children who have been fostered or adopted, this knowledge may not exist, or may be patchy, so it is important to be sensitive to issues around this. Health Visitors use a patient-held record in the UK (the 'red book') to monitor and record early developmental milestones, such as the development of speech, first steps and intermediate steps towards mobility such as 'bottom-shuffling', crawling and toddling. Each of these early milestones gives a range of indicators as whether physical development is progressing in what would be considered a normal pattern. If parents still have their child's red book, this can be a good memory jogger.

Broadly speaking physical development is measured by looking at gross motor skills, the larger muscle movements, and fine motor skills, the smaller muscle movements, that enable smoother manipulation of the body (fingers, etc.). The main developmental milestones that would normally be looked for are summarized in the table below:

Age	Gross motor skills	Fine motor skills
3 months	Learns to support own head	Plays with own hands
6 months	Rolls over independently	Can grasp using whole hand
9 months	Sits up independently and may start crawling	Starts to grasp with pincer action (finger and thumb)
12 months	Able to stand unsupported and may take first steps	Grasp now includes thumb and two or more fingers
15 months	Able to walk independently	Can stack two bricks
2 years	Can run and climb stairs	Stacks multiple bricks in towers
3 years	Confident in manoeuvring and can catch a ball	Able to grasp crayon and draw a basic face
4 years	Able to balance and control a tricycle	Can manage buttons and stack large numbers of bricks
5 years	Climbs, hops and skips	Able to use pencils and colour neatly

Other developmental milestones can be less physically determined, and may be less reliable, so there are much more socially determined elements to feeding practices and independent toileting, for example, which may be culturally determined or subject to the whims of fashion.

The advantage of working in the UK system is that it is broadly supportive of the early development of children, and does have a good paediatric backup system which should mean that all children have been in contact with initially midwives, then Health Visitors who monitor up to the age of five, so parents will generally be aware of whether their children gave any cause for alarm in the early stages. Most parents, for example, will be able to tell you if their children were walking and talking at around the 'normal' times. The system of Community Paediatricians gives a holistic approach to dealing with young people's physical ill health, and their expertise in physical development usually means that any early difficulties should have been addressed and that records of this will exist. Bellman et al. (2013) give a good summary of screening tools and 'red flags' for referral to community paediatricians. The UK system is not, of course, faultless, and there are issues of neglect and deliberate ill-treatment where children have been kept away from this system, so a CAMHS assessment needs to bear this in mind and have a safeguarding element in mind. Rare syndromes of adult mental health, such as factitious illness, where a parent or carer presents frequently with a child who has vague and undetermined physical symptoms, should also be kept in mind if there is an extensive history which seems suspicious. Formerly known as 'Munchausen's syndrome by proxy' this is a difficult issue to deal with from a safeguarding perspective, but should be kept in mind as the potential for both physical and emotional harm to the child is high. In recent years, Safeguarding Children procedures have also started to monitor more closely parents who do not bring their children for hospital and community healthcare appointments as being an indicator of potential neglect (Powell and Appleton 2012).

Whilst being wary of potential safeguarding issues, it is also important to remember also that the concept of 'diagnostic overshadowing' can blind healthcare workers to looking for underlying physical issues as a potential cause for the presenting problems. As nurses in particular we should be conscious of a holistic approach to health. Diagnostic overshadowing is a concept developed in adult mental health and learning disabilities which suggests that an obvious learning disability or mental health history may mean that clinicians assume that this long-standing presentation is the reason for a current issue, and overlook normal investigations that they would have started if the long-standing issues weren't present (Nash 2013). So people with learning disabilities or mental health issues can have their reports of physical pain written off as 'hysterical' or fabricated without a full investigation being completed. This can apply also in children and young people, so it is important to ensure that organic or physical causes for symptoms aren't ignored. This is more obvious in young people presenting with anorexia, for example, where it is important to ask 'Is this purely a psychological issue, or is there another reason for a change in eating patterns?' Nash (ibid) makes the very good argument that this practice of being wary of diagnostic overshadowing is very much in the tradition of non-judgemental practice, itself an essential part of nursing practice. Yet this is in contrast with

Safeguarding practices where we have to be respectful of the choices that people make and understanding of the reasons for their behaviour, but essentially we are making judgements about what needs to be acted upon in line with Safeguarding Children principles. The exercise of clinical judgement for nurses in CAMHS requires us to have enough knowledge of physical healthcare and normal physical development to make these decisions and act upon what we see, to protect vulnerable children and young people.

Box 3.1 Physical Development and Implications for CAMH Nursing
- Parents will normally remember a basic physical developmental history that can help to eliminate physical causes for mental health presentations.
- Young people seen on their own may question the relevance of this, and prefer to concentrate on the current presenting symptoms, in which case follow their lead, and return to this issue later.
- Be aware of Safeguarding (Child Protection) issues when taking a developmental history.
- Physical or organic reasons for presenting symptoms should be considered, and clinicians should be wary of 'diagnostic overshadowing'.

3.3   Cognitive and Emotional Development

Whilst physical development of children and young people is broadly understood and agreed upon, their cognitive development is much more the subject of theorization, and there is much less consensus as to what constitutes 'normal' cognitive development. This, and the fact that young people develop in very individualized ways, makes it much harder to be clear about what elements are important, and often some theoretical models will fit individual circumstances better than others. For fostered and adopted children, for example, issues around attachment may be the most important part of understanding their situation, whilst for others issues around identity or personality formation may make more sense of their situation. For this reason we need to have a broad understanding of different theories in order to be able to apply them to individual needs (see Keenan et al. 2016). The theorists examined below are the principle ones, but there are many more, so we have necessarily had to be selective.

3.3.1   Piaget's Four-Stage Theory

Jean Piaget's (1936) theory is one of the best known concepts of cognitive development and depends on the idea of active learning, that children respond to their environment and adapt to that stimulation. His theories developed from observational studies of a relatively small number of children in his native Switzerland, but have been extensively critiqued and analysed, so the literature on his ideas is quite extensive. Essential to the active learning process is the idea of 'schemas', a conceptualization of how children make sense of the world. These schemas become the building blocks for understanding, so, from a mental health perspective, if these schemas become very fixed and unable to deal with new information or adapt to new situations then distress can occur. Piaget explained this in terms of three phases involved in changing understanding:

- *Assimilation*—where an existing schema is used to understand a new experience.
- *Accommodation*—where an existing schema does not fit the new experience, discovery or knowledge, and needs to be changed to make sense of this new situation.
- *Equilibration*—this is the process of coping when new information cannot be easily accommodated into the existing schemas. An unsettling period of re-examining existing ways of thinking and making sense of the new information. This explains why development may not be a smooth process, as these episodes call for a big leap in understanding.

Piaget therefore proposed a four-stage process, which generally has ages attached to each stage, but this has been critiqued as being too rigid, and even Piaget admitted that, despite the fact that he added age guides to each stage, the process can be much more flexible than this:

- *Sensorimotor stage* (Birth–2 years)
- Infants use their motor skills to explore the world and learn from it. They learn 'Object Permanence', that an object still exists even if they can no longer see it, which requires the ability to make a mental representation of an object.
- *Pre-operational stage* (2–7 years)
- During this stage there is less reliance on physical senses, but they remain 'illogical' thinkers in many ways. Thinking becomes more symbolic, understanding that a word or object can stand for something other than itself. At this stage, children are still egocentric and struggle to see the world from anything other than their own perspective.
- *Concrete operational stage* (7–11 years)
- The development of 'logical' (or operational) thought, which includes working things out internally, though with a concrete representation to help, and a better understanding of abstract concepts like conservation (that quantity may be constant even if appearance changes).
- *Formal operational stage* (11 years and older)

- This stage lasts for the rest of our lives, as we become capable of more abstract thought, and can, for example, test hypotheses to make sense of the world, and make decisions based on the information presented to us.

Box 3.2 Some Implications of Piaget's Theories for Assessment and Understanding

- Piaget thought that children cannot understand the permanence of death until the concrete operational stage, so helping children who have suffered bereavements will be different depending on their age.
- Likewise if they cannot understand the permanence of death, expressing a wish to die themselves (however distressing this is to those around them) is different in younger children than it is for young people who DO understand what it is they are wishing for.
- Younger children who talk about 'hearing voices', but have not yet developed a fuller understanding of external points of view are more likely to reflecting their own internal thinking processes.

3.3.2 Vygotsky's Social Development Theory

Whilst Piaget largely saw development as individual, Lev Vygotsky's (1978) emphasis is much more on the influence of a child's surroundings. He put much more emphasis on culture, surroundings and in particular the role of the adults around the child in development. He also gave more weight to the development of language as an indicator of understanding, saying that whilst thought and language develop initially separately they merge at around the age of three and become intertwined at that point.

The cultural and societal influences in Vygotsky's thought are essential for fostering and guiding cognitive development. This is illustrated in his concept of the *Zone of Proximal Development* which puts the individual child at the centre, effectively what a child can learn on their own, but then has the surrounding zone expanding the potential for learning through the influence of 'knowledgeable others' (parents, family, neighbours, teachers and peers) and technology and tools. These provide the scaffolding that guides learning, though inevitably this will have a cultural bias and be limited by the interests and bias of the knowledgeable others. Beyond this zone is an area which is initially out of reach, but which the individual can access as they become more independent, and potentially less constricted by their immediate surroundings. This obviously has implications for educational theory and guided learning as well as peer-based collaborative learning.

The emphasis Vygotsky put on language development also provided a staged understanding of cognitive development based on the idea that language is the primary method for adults to communicate ideas to children. He saw language in four forms:

- *Primitive speech*, from birth to around 2 years, consisting of single words or phrases, largely imitative or expressing basic emotions.

- *Social speech*, or a naïve psychological stage, from around 2 to 4 years, when we use communicate with each other, and the fascination with the names of objects illustrates an understanding of symbolism.
- *Private speech*, generally from age 4 to 7 years, essentially saying out loud what you are thinking as you think it, which serves an intellectual processing and self-regulating function.
- *Inner speech*, from age 8 when the private speech becomes internal thought with no need for vocalization.

Box 3.3 Vygotsky's Social Development Theory Applied

Vygotsky illustrates well the link between how people think and what they say. By tuning into how children and young people phrase their thoughts we have a good chance to see how those ideas have developed, and how we can help them to overcome hurdles in their cognitive processing. CBT and systemic therapies both put a lot of emphasis on how language is linked to thought and use this as a way of challenging unhelpful thinking, and looking for alternative ways of understanding feelings and emotions.

Although Vygotsky emphasizes the positives of social and cultural influences, these can also be limiting, and presenting alternative ways of thinking about the world beyond that to which some children and young people have been acclimatized by virtue of their upbringing can lead to some challenging discussions.

3.3.3   Bronfenbrenner's Ecological Systems Theory

Vygotsky was not the only theorist who put emphasis on social aspects of learning and child development, another important figure was Urie Bronfenbrenner (1979) who took a more balanced view of the 'nature versus nurture' debate to develop his systems theory. In broader terms, systemic theory also underpins what used to be called 'Family Therapy' but is now usually referred to as systemic psychotherapy.

Although Bronfenbrenner's work has been primarily influential in early years education (Hayes et al. 2017), it is also useful to keep in mind through the whole range of young people, as the societal and systemic influences shift and change as young people develop more independence from their families and instead become more reliant on peer group interactions and wider social influences. Bronfenbrenner's original model proposes five concentric circles surrounding the individual (though he later developed the bioecological model which puts more emphasis on the role that individual health, including the genetic basis of individuals, is likely to contribute, thus evening up the 'nature' element of 'nature versus nurture').

- *Microsystem* is the most immediate surroundings to the individual, usually family initially, but also including local school, local faith group, healthcare workers and peers.
- *Mesosystem* includes the complex interactions between different elements of the microsystem, focused on the quality of those interactions and the influence they have on the individual.
- *Exosystem* widens out to those elements of society which influence those around the individual, including healthcare and social care systems, parental workplaces, politics and media influence on the beliefs of those immediately involved.
- *Macrosystem* includes the broadest influences acting on the individual, ethnicity, socio-economic status, common cultural values, identity and heritage.
- *Chronosystem* is a final influence which doesn't fit easily with the two-dimensional concentric circle model but recognizes the way that these factors will change over the lifespan, and particularly will become disrupted at times of transition.

Box 3.4 Bronfenbrenner and Systemic Thinking
- This model illustrates the social influences which act in a systemic manner on individuals, and builds on the 'nurture' element that suggests we are all products of our environment, even if our reactions to that environment may change over time.
- Systemic psychotherapy (family therapy) uses similar thinking in developing therapeutic approaches to family difficulties.
- These ideas are particularly important for younger children who are very dependent for all their needs on those around them and develop in reaction to those surroundings. Older young people may choose to reject some of these values and develop more individual agency and independence.

3.3.4 The Psychoanalysts: Sigmund Freud, Anna Freud and Melanie Klein

Psychoanalytic theory has proven to be controversial, and it has not found widespread use within contemporary child mental health. There are one or two exceptions in the application of child psychotherapy and art psychotherapies, though are both underfunded and relatively uncommon resources, at least within the National Health Service. Psychoanalysis has, however, given us some important concepts which need to noted as they have entered popular thinking.

Sigmund Freud's work was important (alongside that of Jung) in developing the concept of a conscious and unconscious mind, essentially those things that we think clearly about, and those thoughts and feelings which we may not have so much clarity about where they are coming from, but are a powerful part of our emotional reactions. Freud's work on the development of personality during childhood (his theory was that personality is essentially fixed at quite an early age, around 5 years old) revolved around a series of stages at which it was possible to get stuck or fixated, and which may need to be returned to repair damage if those stages are not correctly negotiated. The psychosexual development stages, oral, anal, phallic, latent and genital, have been extensively critiqued since Freud first suggested them, from a variety of angles. Scientifically his reliance on individual case studies rather than empirical positivist research suggests that attempts to generalize meaning from such a small sample go against what we would now regard as rigorous research methodologies. His interpretations of these case studies are grounded in the inherent bias of his own situation and largely address male heterosexuality rather than female aspects of development, for example.

Anna Freud, Sigmund's youngest daughter, made her own contribution to psychoanalysis with her identification of 'defence mechanisms' and went on to develop a better understanding of the use of psychoanalysis with children and young people. Whilst she remained essentially true to her father's core thinking, Anna Freud applied psychoanalysis to a practical psychotherapy for younger people (Sigmund Freud only records one case of a younger person, 'Little Hans'). Anna Freud's work emphasized the use of therapeutic alliance, and treating young people as individuals, joining them at whatever level they were able to work, whilst exploring the meaning of what they were doing.

Melanie Klein further developed the discipline of child psychotherapy, largely based on Anna Freud's work, but with more emphasis on the first year of life, with the theory that this was the critical period in which all future psychological reactions were determined. The unconscious phantasy that she suggested developed during this period pre-determined future reactions, and it is from this that she developed 'Object Relations Theory'. This theory (based on Freudian psychoanalysis) suggests that young children develop an internalized relationship with not just objects but their primary caretakers (usually the mother) and that these relationships determine all future reactions and relationships. The potential for this to become very blaming of mothers has been widely critiqued. Whilst she was not alone in this (Bowlby made similar mistakes, as we will see), it did contribute to an atmosphere of blaming parents that has not been helpful in engaging parents ever since.

Other creative therapies have developed from the psychoanalytic tradition. Play therapy is an effective way of engaging younger children who struggle to verbalize or articulate their difficulties, and the Jungian-based tradition of art psychotherapies can be very effective with some young people. Likewise drama therapies can be a good way to engage young people who struggle with more traditional psychotherapeutic interventions. Sadly the lack of a robust evidence-base disadvantages these therapies in the competition for NHS funds, so they have been increasingly squeezed out of commissioned services and are more commonly found as private or third sector provision, which means that not all children and young people can access them.

Box 3.5 The Influence of Psychoanalysis
- Psychoanalysis was a major part of twentieth century thinking and introduced several concepts which we now take for granted as part of the understanding of the human condition, despite the lack of a scientific basis for the theories.
- Anna Freud and Melanie Klein developed psychoanalytic child psychotherapy, which still has a place in the treatment of some young people, but is a rare resource in the NHS.
- Other forms of creative therapies, each with distinct trainings and applications, have grown out of this tradition and provide a good therapeutic avenue for children and young people who struggle to verbalize their feelings and emotions.

3.3.5   Beyond Psychoanalysis: Erikson

Erik Erikson is generally described as a psychoanalyst (Schlein 2016), but his work moved beyond the Freudian and Jungian traditions into a full formed psychosocial theory of development which covered the whole life cycle. Erikson argues that his model is a tool or framework to help understand the human condition and that each stage contains a crisis of some kind which must be met and the outcome of that crisis determines the progress of the next part of the journey. Of these the phrase 'identity crisis' is the best known in popular culture. We will look at just the first five stages which take us to age 18 in his schema, though arguably the sixth stage, of intimacy versus isolation, which covers the period dominated by adult intimate relations, should also be considered. As an aside, given Erikson's focus on crises, the term 'mid-life crisis' does not belong to him, but was actually coined by another psychoanalyst, Elliott Jaques.

Trust vs. mistrust (0–18 months). In the presence of a consistent caregiver, the infant learns to develop trust in those around him, and this trust is transferable to others. The absence of a relationship of this kind will foreshadow longer term issues of mistrust and uncertainty in future relationships where it is hard to give or accept trust. This stage is the basis of Bowlby's work which we will cover next.

Autonomy vs. shame and doubt (18–36 months). During this stage, children develop a sense of independence and free will and need to be encouraged to do more and more for themselves, rather than relying on adults for everything. This fosters a sense of self-esteem and achievement which feeds into confidence levels.

Initiative vs. guilt (3–5 years). Characterized by interactive play with peers at school the task of leading play, or co-operating together, is primary. Children who fail to take any initiative will feel guilt which again will impact on their personality development.

Industry vs. Inferiority (5–12 years). Children become more dependent on their peer group than on parents and either develop industrious feelings of competence or start to feel failure and develop feelings of inferiority. Again these feelings are likely to affect their ongoing development. Social pressures to demonstrate ability in one or more areas become more prominent, so self-perception is likely to be affected by either successes or failures, and reactions to those events.

Identity vs. role confusion (12–18). An adolescent preoccupation develops as the young person separates from their family emotionally and seeks their place as an independent person in their own right. This 'identity crisis' includes a period of exploration as the young person seeks to find what works for them and what doesn't, and will include an understanding of their own sexuality, for example. It can include a rebellion against what they have been taught or what they perceive as being expected of them.

Box 3.6 Erikson's Stages of Life
- Erikson's concept of adolescent identity crisis has much face validity in trying to understand the difficulties we see in young people.
- The strong need to understand themselves and their place in life (alongside some physical hormonal changes) can be a very distressing time for young people. Separating out normal experimentation and exploration from illness and danger of harm can be difficult for clinicians and parents alike.
- Trying to meet the expectations of others around them (to achieve academically, or conform to cultural norms, for example) whilst having different ideas about what they want for themselves can lead to self-harming or destructive behaviours in the absence of other coping mechanisms.
- For many adolescents, trying to make sense of the conflicting demands on them means this is the most difficult part of their lives, and the stigma (and sometimes difficulty) of accessing help as well as a misplaced idea that they are old enough to cope without help can lead to reluctance to seek advice. Likewise young people may be vulnerable to malicious advice (online or from peers) or to seeking identity within gang cultures.

3.3.6 Bowlby's Attachment Theory

John Bowlby defined attachment as a lasting psychological attachment between human beings, and his trilogy of books (1968, 1973, 1980) have had a lasting effect on how we understand the idea of bonding between humans. Initially developed as a way of understanding the bond between (primarily) mother and child, it was later extended to take into account relationships between adults. Bowlby's work was set in post-war Britain and has been criticized for the emphasis it puts on the maternal bond rather than taking into account the paternal role in Western societies. More broadly different cultural models also take a more community-based approach to child-rearing rather than seeing it as a function of a single nuclear family, so this does not sit easily with these ideas. The phrase 'maternal deprivation', for example, is very blaming and can be seen as putting undue pressure on mothers to conform to socially constructed norms. John Bowlby's theories had several main points:

- A newborn child has an inborn need for one main attachment figure, a concept known as monotropy. Bowlby didn't contest that other attachments are important too, but stresses that a single main attachment of a consistent nature was vital.
- This attachment should be unbroken for the first 2 years of life, and that absence of this consistent attachment (maternal deprivation) would have long-term consequences.
- Long-term consequences of maternal deprivation could include aggression, delinquency, reduced intelligence, depression and even affectionless psychopathy.
- Even short-term separation from the main attachment figure could lead to distress characterized by protest, despair and detachment.
- The nature of the attachment shapes the development of the child's internal model for understanding relationships and in the longer term guides the understanding of how trustworthy others can be, as well as determining self-perception and worth.

From this Bowlby and others determined various types of attachment: secure attachments, anxious-ambivalent attachments, anxious-avoidant attachments, and disorganized or disoriented attachments. The aim of good parenting therefore becomes to provide this 'secure base' (Bowlby 1990).

The clinical application of these theories have primarily been in understanding difficulties in fostering and adoption relationships (i.e. Schofield and Beek 2018), but there are some dangers in using the term too freely (as well as the criticisms of the underlying theory). The overlap of symptoms with some of the features of autism spectrum disorder (ASD) means that caution needs to be used, and a thorough assessment completed to avoid mixing up the two conditions (McKenzie and Dallos 2017).

Box 3.7 Application of Bowlby's Attachment Theories
- Bowlby's theories have been extensively critiqued and need to be used with caution in order to maintain a non-judgemental stance, but they can be useful in some situations.
- In particular the overlap of presentation with autism spectrum disorder means a careful differential diagnostic assessment is made in order to ensure that the correct course of treatment can be determined.

3.4 Adverse Childhood Experiences (ACEs) as a Concept Informing Treatments

In adult mental health, a better understanding of trauma informed treatments along with advances in the clinical neurosciences has changed how adult treatments are developing (i.e. Gianfrancesco et al. 2019). This is starting to have some effect in the way that we think about treating young people too, as a review by Black et al. (2012) demonstrated. A lot of the impetus for this understanding came from the original study into Adverse Childhood Experiences (ACEs) conducted in San Diego (Fellitti et al. 1998). This study demonstrated a link between these early experiences and consequent coping mechanisms which may be maladaptive, and poor outcomes for health in the long term, and has strongly influenced psychological thinking since it was first published. Boullier and Blair (2018) have summarized also how ACEs impact on physical health and development, and survey work completed by Public Health Wales (PHW 2015) has demonstrated the extent to which ACEs can be seen to affect the population.

Adverse childhood experiences, as defined by the original study, cover a range of different experiences:

- *Abuse*: physical, emotional and sexual
- *Household Challenges*: mother treated violently, household substance abuse, mental illness in household, parental separation or divorce, and criminal household member (involving imprisonment)
- *Neglect*: emotional neglect and physical neglect

This wide range of experiences are identified as having potentially cumulative effects on children and young people so the more of these experiences there are during childhood the more likely it is that the effects will be adverse in terms of physical or mental health. A public health preventative approach has been used in some areas, particularly the family nurse partnership scheme, which aims to improve health behaviours in families, but this understanding of the impact of ACEs on health has also informed treatment approaches (i.e. Hunt et al. 2017). Perhaps the most important impact that our improved understanding of ACEs has had in is emphasizing the degree to which children and young people are affected by what is going on around them, that they are actively affected by this, not just unaffected witnesses (Callaghan et al. 2018).

Box 3.8 Adverse Childhood Experiences
- The concept of ACEs takes a range of childhood experiences and emphasizes the degree to which these impact on children and young people's mental and physical health into adulthood.
- Families will often be reluctant to talk about some of these events, and it may be difficult to elicit vital information which clearly has an impact on helping to find new coping mechanisms and provide healthier ways of living.
- ACEs emphasize the degree to which experiences of a variety of negative experiences can impact health, drawing on an extensive body of evidence.

3.5   Development of Resilience as a Way of Understanding Coping

Another concept which informs development and treatment is that of resilience. This is based on the observation that people seem to react differently to similar experiences, some seem to cope well, whilst others have very negative reactions. Not all veterans who experience war-zone traumatic experiences develop post-traumatic stress disorder, for example, despite having been through exactly the same circumstances. Emmy Werner is credited with the first application of the term resilience in this context, based on a longitudinal study of different outcomes for deprived children in Hawaii in 1971 (reported in Werner and Smith 1982). She noted that whilst many of the children in the same area, with the same experiences, were badly effected, a significant proportion were not. This has led to subsequent studies which have increased our understanding of 'protective factors', positive behaviours or coping mechanisms, or character traits which allow some people to thrive when others do less well. Increasing the positive elements, therefore, can not only be a predictor of who will survive adverse experiences better, but can also allow changes to thinking and behaving, often employing techniques from cognitive behavioural approaches, which increase resilience and enable either better coping or recovery.

The concept of protective factors is complex, but as summarized by Zolkoski and Bullock (2012) as including the following elements:

- Individual factors: such as supportive caring relationships and a positive outlook on life
- Self-regulation: an ability to cope with emotional setbacks and confidence in overcoming hurdles and setbacks
- Self-concept: particularly an attitude that sees hardships as learning experiences on which to build
- Family support: responsive warm parents or carers who can provide a warm and loving environment which allows stimulation and new experiences
- Community support: good relationships within the community, including faith communities

Other systems of understanding protective factors will stress more specific things, like having an ability which makes you stand out (be it football or a sporting 'talent', playing an instrument, or a particular expertise or interest in one topic).

This understanding of building healthier young people, both physically and mentally, has obvious implications for public health, and the emphasis on prevention has made it a popular topic. The UK government, for example, includes a section on this on its Mentally Healthy Schools website: https://www.mentallyhealthyschools.org.uk/

3.6 Issues of Neurodevelopmental Disorders and Learning Disabilities

As we noted above, there is a potential danger of misdiagnosis when symptoms can be interpreted in different ways. Autism spectrum disorders can be difficult to detect, and whilst Community Paediatricians will screen and diagnose many cases at a young age it is increasingly common for young people in their teenage years to attend community CAMHS and be diagnosed with ASD (after a thorough assessment) rather than primarily with a mental health issue. Ozonoff et al. (2018) have examined this phenomenon of late or delayed diagnosis in the US, and Bargiela et al. (2016) have illustrated some of the issues relating to autism presenting differently in women, and the effects this can have in delaying the diagnostic process.

Likewise it is important to recognize that children and young people with learning or intellectual disabilities may not respond to any of the screening tools, or many of the developmental systems in the same ways as those without these disadvantages. Learning problems will usually be diagnosed by the Community Paediatricians, but, as with the neurodevelopmental issues, it is possible for children and young people to slip through the net and not have formal diagnoses, but still have significant unmet needs, which will need assessment and referral for more detailed assessment if necessary. Diagnostic overshadowing works in different directions, so assuming a mental health issue is the root cause of presenting symptoms when they may be better explained by a learning disability is also a possibility.

With both these areas, and with physical disability, it is important to remember that comorbidities occur frequently, and untangling them can be difficult (see Rhagavan et al. 2011). Young people with autism are frequently very anxious, for example, or frustrated by their inability to understand what is expected of them by those around them, and may react in ways which are hard for 'neurotypical' people to comprehend. Young people with physical disability can become depressed, anxious or psychotic like their able-bodied peers, and children and young people with learning disabilities suffer from mental health difficulties on top of their other disadvantages.

3.7 Summary

This has necessarily been a brief look at some of the most important theories informing the practice of child and young people's mental health. Space prevents us looking at the important work of major figures like Bettelheim, Skinner, Winnicott, Bandura and others. Likewise the study of the development of personality is often separated out and we have not addressed this as a discrete issue, even though it is important for the concept of 'emerging undiagnosed personality disorders' which are sometimes discussed in child and adolescent mental health circles.

What is most important for nurses to bear in mind is that children and young people are still developing. Some of their issues will be about not yet having developed coping mechanisms for difficult emotional experiences, or traumatic situations. Whilst in adult mental health the concept of recovery is important, children and young people are not necessarily recovering to a stable position, they are still developing towards a place where they are able to cope with what life throws at them. Consequently our attempts at therapeutic intervention need to take account of where they each are, individually, and what can be expected of them, and what help they need to manage the next stage of their journey.

References

Bargiela S, Steward R, Mandy W (2016) The experiences of late diagnosed women with autism spectrum conditions: an investigation of the female autism phenotype. J Autism Dev Disord 46:3281–3294

Bellman M, Byrne O, Sege R (2013) BMJ clinical review: developmental assessment of children. Br Med J 346:e8687

Black JB, Woodworth M, Tremblay M, Carpenter T (2012) A review of trauma-informed treatment for adolescents. Can Psychol 53(3):192–203

Boullier M, Blair M (2018) Adverse childhood experiences. Paediatr Child Health 28:3

Bowlby J (1968) Attachment and loss: Vol. 1. Attachment. Basic Books, New York

Bowlby J (1973) Attachment and loss: Vol. 2 separation anxiety and anger. Penguin Books, London

Bowlby J (1980) Attachment and loss: Vol. 3 loss, sadness and depression. Basic Books, New York

Bowlby J (1990) A secure base: parent-child attachment and human development. Basic Books, New York

Bronfenbrenner U (1979) The ecology of human development: experiments by nature and design. Harvard University Press, Cambridge

Callaghan JEM, Alexander JH, Sixsmith J, Fellin LC (2018) Beyond 'witnessing': children's experiences of coercive control in domestic violence and abuse. J Interpers Violence 33(10):1551–1581

Fellitti VJ, Anda RF, Nordenburg D, Williamson DF, Spitz AM, Edwards V, Koss MP, Marks JS (1998) Relationship of childhood abuse and household dysfunction to many of the leading causes of death in adulthood: the adverse childhood experiences (ACE) study. Am J Prev Med 14(4):245–258

Gianfrancesco O, Bubb VJ, Quinn JP (2019) Transforming the "E" in "G x E": trauma-informed approaches and psychological therapy interventions in psychosis. Front Psych 10:9

Hayes N, O'Toole L, Halpenny AM (2017) Introducing Bronfenbrenner: (introducing early years thinkers series). Routledge, London

Hunt KA, Slack KS, Berger LM (2017) Adverse childhood experiences and behavioral problems in middle childhood. Child Abuse Negl 67:391–402

Keenan T, Evans S, Crowley K (2016) An introduction to child development (sage foundations of psychology series). Sage Publications, London

McKenzie R, Dallos R (2017) Autism and attachment difficulties: overlap of symptoms, implications and innovative solutions. Clin Child Psychol Psychiatry 22(4):632–648

Mercer J (2018) Child development: concepts and theories. Sage Publications, London

Nash M (2013) Diagnostic overshadowing: a potential barrier to physical healthcare for mental health service users. Ment Health Pract 17(4):22–26

Ozonoff S, Young GS, Brian J, Charman T, Shephard E, Solish A, Zweigenbaum L (2018) Diagnosis of autism spectrum disorder after age 5 in children evaluated longitudinally since infancy. J Am Acad Child Adolesc Psychiatry 57(11):849–857

Piaget J (1936) Origins of intelligence in the child. Routledge and Keegan Paul, London

Powell C, Appleton JV (2012) Children and young people's missed healthcare appointments: reconceptualising 'did not attend' to 'was not brought'—a review of the evidence for practice. J Res Nurs 17(2):181–192

Public Health Wales (2015) Welsh adverse childhood experiences (ACE) study: adverse childhood experiences and their effect on health-harming behaviours in the welsh adult population. PHW, Cardiff

Rhagavan R, Bernard S, McCarthy J (2011) Mental health needs of children and Young people with learning disabilities. Pavilion Publishing, Brighton

Schlein S (2016) The clinical Erik Erikson. Routledge, London

Schofield G, Beek M (2018) Attachment handbook for fostering and adoption, 2nd edn. CoramBAAF, London

Vygotsky LS (1978) Mind in society: the development of higher psychological processes. Harvard University Press, Cambridge

Werner E, Smith RS (1982) Vulnerable but invincible: a longitudinal study of resilient children and youth. McGraw Hill, New York

Zolkoski SM, Bullock LM (2012) Resilience in children and youth: a review. Child Youth Serv Rev 34(12):2295–2303

Useful Websites

MindEd E-learning resource (includes developmental resources). https://www.minded.org.uk/

US Centre for Disease Control—Child Development section. https://www.cdc.gov/ncbddd/child-development/index.html

UK Mumsnet pages on Child Development (up to age 5). https://www.mumsnet.com/babies/child-development

World Health Organization Child Development Pages. https://www.who.int/topics/early-child-development/en/

Chapter 4
Nursing Children and Young People in Specialist CAMHS Inpatient Settings

Tim McDougall

4.1 Introduction

Inpatient care for children and young people is defined as a specialist service (NHS England 2018). Many chapters about care for children and young people in other such services such as cancer, cardiac or respiratory provision begin with a clear summary of what they are, why they exist and who they are for. It is almost impossible to apply this formula in a chapter about inpatient CAMHS. First of all, relatively little is written about hospital admission for children and young people with mental health problems, and much of that is based on anecdote and opinion rather than on robust evidence. The research base for the efficacy of inpatient treatment is limited for most, if not all, mental disorders affecting children and young people (Cotgrove 2013).

Secondly, historical accounts vary widely and are often contradictory. Many are steeped in the discourse of psychiatry, psychology or sociology, and parochial differences play out which can become a distraction from the debate about the role and purpose of inpatient units (see Cottrell and Kraam 2005; Williams and Kerfoot 2005). Differences in philosophy and language between agencies and the professions have sometimes made multidisciplinary and multi-agency working difficult (Wolpert et al. 2014), which in turn has limited the quality and breadth of the evidence.

Thirdly, UK national policy on which to guide commissioners, providers and professionals in relation to care in the inpatient setting has been haphazard and lacking in ambition rather than strategy for over two decades (see House of Commons Health Committee 1997; Department of Health 2014; National Audit Office 2018; House of Commons Library 2019). The debate about what to do to help young

T. McDougall (✉)
Greater Manchester Mental Health NHS Foundation Trust, Manchester, UK
e-mail: Tim.McDougall@gmmh.nhs.uk

© Springer Nature Switzerland AG 2020
L. Baldwin (ed.), *Nursing Skills for Children and Young People's Mental Health*,
https://doi.org/10.1007/978-3-030-18679-1_4

people in mental health crisis has almost exclusively been about beds or the perceived lack of these (Hillen and Szaniecki 2010; Myers et al. 2018). Future in Mind is the latest of several long-term policies that aim to improve mental health outcomes for children and young people (Department of Health 2015). Although this has provided some additional investment and raised the profile of mental health, there has been little attention to inpatient care and the main political focus of the current government to date has been on schools as part of the so-called 2020 Reforms (Department for Education 2018).

Together these issues amount to a poorly informed and confused picture regarding inpatient CAMHS. The available literature fails to answer the question of who may benefit from inpatient admission and who should do what to help. This chapter does not attempt to categorically answer these questions and provide a definitive position on why inpatient CAMHS exists. Nor does it attempt to delineate the exclusive role nurses play in CAMHS which has sometimes been about carving out territory as the separate disciplines seek to make sense of their own individual professional contributions rather than focus on the sum of the parts. Instead, this chapter offers another perspective which in time will form part of the rich but often confusing tapestry of the literature, which may or may not help clarify the future role and function of CAMHS inpatient care.

4.2   History of Inpatient Care

Residential care, confinement and treatment have long been part of the public response to the perceived needs of mentally ill, handicapped, homeless and deviant children (Parry-Jones 1998). The origins of inpatient CAMHS go back to eighteenth century poor houses of the United States (US) and workhouses of the United Kingdom (UK). The Lunacy Act of 1845 was a key milestone, affecting people with a whole spectrum of needs. Following passage of this, children with mental health, learning disability or general development needs could be transferred from local workhouses to institutions or county asylums. Case reports refer to children being frightened by dogs or being tossed by cows, non-appearance of menses and cutting of teeth as reasons for admission. Dangerous or suicidal children might be given bromide, chloroform or brandy in an attempt to manage, contain or cure them Gingell (2001).

A notable landmark in the history of inpatient CAMHS was the opening of Great Ormond Street Hospital in London in 1852. In his lectures between 1845 and 1860, Charles West, the founder of the hospital, spoke of hypochondriasis, night terrors and disorders of the highest function of the brain. Walk (1964) wrote that treatment for such conditions affecting children was separation from parents or boarding with a quiet family. Today, Great Ormond Street offers inpatient CAMHS for children with eating disorders and other mental health conditions. Parents are actively encouraged to visit rather than stay away from their children, which is a change in attitudes informed by attachment theory (see Bowlby 1951). This has not only influenced hospital child visiting policies, but has also positively informed institutional care, child custody and maternal employment.

Another landmark was the opening of the Royal Albert Hospital in Lancaster in 1870. This was originally called the '*Royal Albert Asylum for the Care, Education and Training of Idiots, Imbeciles and Weak Minded Children and Young Person's of the Northern Counties*'. This is an early illustration of the confusion between mental disorder and learning disability which to some extent remains today. Today, the Royal Albert Hospital has evolved to become an Islamic education centre for Muslim girls, which shows how the passage of time sees changes in attitudes towards children.

In the 1940s, inpatient psychiatric units for children began to open in England. This coincided with the introduction of approved schools and borstals for delinquent children, but this was not part of any coordinated political response to the distinct needs of children. The first CAMHS inpatient units were modelled on the residential communities of the US and were mainly custodial in their aim and function. It was only later that these were to become therapeutically orientated and focused on what Cameron (1949) coined the socio-psychobiological unity of the child. There followed a rapid expansion of adolescent units until the 1980s when the concept of the 'general purpose' inpatient unit was introduced. Children and young people could be admitted for short- and long-term care as well as in an emergency (NHS Health Advisory Service 1985).

Most inpatient CAMHS units functioning during the 1980s operated along the lines of therapeutic communities and placed a strong emphasis on the therapeutic milieu. Twenty to thirty years ago they were often led by charismatic leaders with idiosyncratic operational policies. With little evidence base to guide them, therapeutic practice was determined by the varied experience of the staff, but often focusing on long-term therapeutic interventions for children and young people with complex needs rather than those with serious mental illness such as psychosis (Cotgrove 2013).

In the years that followed a number of high profile scandals exposed failings in the care and treatment of children, many of whom had mental health problems and disorders. The so-called '*Pindown Scandal*' of the 1980s exposed the restrictive practice of staff in a number of children's homes in Staffordshire. The practice of isolating, restraining and humiliating children was condemned as unethical, unprofessional and illegal (Levy and Kahan 1991). Such practice has not yet been eradicated completely as various Care Quality Commission (CQC) reports of inpatient CAMHS have highlighted (CQC 2018). Problems with overly restrictive child care have not been unique to the UK. Indeed, most research into the restraint or restriction of liberty of children and young people in mental health settings has been undertaken in the US (Wilson et al. 2015). Weiss (1990) reported on children who had died as a result of physical and mechanical restraint in the care of US public institutions. Many died of asphyxiation due to chest compression during restraint. Weiss' influential report promoted far reaching regulations to prevent, reduce and monitor physical restraint (Masters 2017), and some of this has crossed the water to be reflected in British policy including the current focus on reducing prone restraint.

Just as interesting as the background to CAMHS inpatient care is the history of restraint in such settings. This has originated from the juvenile justice sector as well as adult mental health services, which in turn has been influenced by the practice in prisons and secure hospitals. A legal precedent for the use of restraint was established with the English vagrancy laws of the 1700s (Masters 2017) and there is much documented evidence of use throughout the ages (Mind 2013). The infamous 1960s film, *One Flew Over the Cuckoo's Nest*, drew public attention to the use of restriction in mental health settings and played a largely negative role in publicising and propagating stigma and consolidating the role of restraint in mental health. Understanding the principles of least restrictive practice and applying these in day-to-day nursing care is a key part of the inpatient CAMHS nursing role (McDougall and Nolan 2017). The concept of least restriction originated in the US has been described in the international health and social care literature over many years (see Carr et al. 1999; Smith et al. 2005). It is frequently reported in conjunction with nursing practice (Muir-Cochrane et al. 2018) and is enshrined in the Mental Health Code of Practice. The code requires mental health service providers and the practitioners within them to reduce restrictive interventions including restraint, seclusion and rapid tranquillisation. It is nurses who are most commonly involved in restrictive interventions, and so it is nurses who must transform their practice. There are a number of strategies that can support nurses to reduce ward-based conflict, violence and aggression. These include Safewards which is now recognised as an international model of restraint reduction (Bowers 2014).

Derbyshire Safeguarding Children Board (2018) recently published an independent inquiry into the experiences of children and young people at Aston Hall in Derbyshire between the 1950s and 1970s. The report described children being stripped naked, put in straitjackets, drugged and sexually assaulted. Like many of its kind, this so-called treatment centre closed quietly in 2004 which reflected attitudes to care of children in the state at the time. The *Cleveland Inquiry* (Butler-Sloss 1987) and the abuse of children in care in Wales (Department of Health 2000) each highlighted problems that many young people had with their mental health and the use of restriction and physical abuse by staff who were charged with their care. It is possible that other such inquiries will follow, as the ongoing Independent Inquiry into Child Sexual Abuse gives the historical abuse of children in public care, the profile and attention it deserves.

Despite numerous public inquiries into the care and treatment of young people with mental health problems, little changed up until the 1980s when a key report entitled *Bridges Over Troubled Waters* was published (Horrocks 1986). This made recommendations about service models and access. However, it was to be another decade before *Together We Stand* was published by the Health Advisory Service (1995). This recommended that a four-tier model for CAMHS provision was proposed to guide the commissioning, role and management of CAMHS. In the 20 or so years that followed the tiered model failed to give any widespread traction to political or service development and was often conceptually misunderstood (Joint Commissioning Panel for Mental Health 2013). Following publication of *Future in Mind* (Department of Health 2015), there was a move away from this framework towards the Thrive model as part of the current transformation of children and young people's mental health services. Whether this brings some systematic focus to who does what for which young people remains to be seen.

4.3   Inpatient Care Today

Inpatient units for children and young people are commissioned to provide assessment, treatment and crisis care for children and young people with complex, persistent or severe mental disorders (NHSE 2018). However, as practice rather than policy or strategy has determined, factors that lead to inpatient CAMHS admission are not only the acuity or chronicity of the child or young person's mental health difficulties, but also lack of response to community treatment, breakdown in therapeutic relationships and level of risk to self or others.

As with many aspects of specialist CAMHS, the planning of inpatient care has been ad-hoc rather than strategic. This is partly due to the history of commissioning and uncertainty about whether planning should occur locally, regionally or nationally and whether clinicians should be included or excluded in that process. It is generally accepted that the current distribution of inpatient beds is failing to meet need (NHSE 2014; Frith 2017) but whether that means there are too many or too few beds is another matter which is difficult to specify without attention to the wider pathway. In a review of child and adolescent mental health services more generally, the CQC (2017) found a significant mismatch between demand and capacity for inpatient admission. Of course demand is not the same as need, and many argue that most children and young people never require hospital admission.

There is a common misconception that CAMHS care and treatment and hospital admission are synonymous, a widely held belief that has helped maintain the historical neglect in commissioning such services. Use of the terms 'Tier 4' and 'inpatient' are often used interchangeably. The growing media attention on the emotional health and well-being of children and young people has been spuriously linked to a lack of inpatient services. The most recent specifications for commissioning highly specialised services aim to dispel this conceptual misunderstanding by including 'non-admitted care' including crisis intervention, home treatment, step-down care and other alternatives to hospital admission (NHSE 2018). However, access to non-admitted care remains poorly defined and patchy in reality within the commissioned English services and across the wider UK.

These factors combinedly mean that the predominant model of intervention for young people in mental health crisis or with serious mental illness remains one of hospital admission. This is despite evidence that alternatives to admission such as intensive community and day care, outpatient treatment and home-based services can often be more effective, cheaper and acceptable to young people and families (McDougall et al. 2008). Gaps in access to hospital, intensive community and home-based services for children and young people have historically led to care or containment in settings such as paediatric wards, adult mental health wards or police custody (Department of Health and NHS England 2015).

At the time of writing this chapter, inpatient CAMHS is receiving much public attention. Media stories about young people in police cells and children travelling many miles from home to receive hospital care have generated concern about access to help for children and young people in mental health crisis. The rapid increase in young people being admitted to inpatient units or other inappropriate settings has been confirmed in various reviews and reports (McDougall 2014; NHS England 2014; Home Affairs Select Committee 2015). An independent report from the Mental Health Taskforce (2016) was published in response to the Five Year Forward View for Mental Health. This included specific recommendations for children and young people, including ending the practice of sending young people out of their local area for acute inpatient care as soon as possible. Various ministerial statements were to follow, with the latest stating a commitment to eliminate inappropriate placements to inpatient beds for children and young people by 2021 (Prime Minister's Office 2017).

Whilst a range of positive outcomes and user satisfaction have been reported (Jacobs et al. 2004; Tulloch et al. 2008), inpatient mental health care for children and young people has received much public scrutiny and a significant amount of bad press in recent years. The CQC has found many services requiring improvement and some have been judged inadequate or closed. This is because they have been unsafe or because the providers have failed to improve regulated quality standards. The Quality Network for Inpatient CAMHS (QNIC) sets a number of minimum quality and best practice standards that apply directly to registered nurses and the practice of health care assistants or support workers who currently provide the majority of direct care in CAMHS inpatient units. The standards address environment and facilities; staffing and training; access, admission and discharge; care and treatment; information, consent and confidentiality; young people's rights and safeguarding; and clinical governance. The QNIC standards are well regarded both by service providers and commissioners and the CQC and are used within 95% of inpatient units.

In their review of standards of care in CAMHS, the CQC (2017) highlighted safety as their single biggest concern. This included the use of restraint, seclusion and long-term segregation as well as sexual safety and the poor physical environment of many wards. This is interesting since the very fabric of inpatient CAMHS wards is linked to the concept of the therapeutic milieu which is seen as integral to the success of inpatient care. Milieu therapy has been used with children since the late 1800s, when the so-called moral treatment and therapeutic communities were the key approaches in the treatment of choice for psychiatric problems and disorders (Sergeant 2009).

4.4   Nursing Staff and Skill Mix in Inpatient Settings

It is not just the perceived lack of beds and the quality and safety of inpatient care that has been in the media spotlight. The staffing, skill mix and quality of care provided in inpatient child and adolescent mental health services have also been called into question. Nurse recruitment, retention and training have increasingly become significant areas of challenge over the years, and this is just as evident in the CAMHS inpatient setting as it is more generally (NHS England 2014). Multiple high profile reports have confirmed that the number and skill mix of nurses makes a difference to quality of care, patient experience and clinical outcomes (Francis 2013). Care Quality Commission (CQC) standards state that to safeguard people's health, safety and welfare there must be sufficient numbers of suitably qualified, skilled and experienced staff (CQC 2012). This has also been illustrated in various high profile reports of nursing and care staff including the Cavendish Review (Department of Health 2013a, b, c), the Berwick Review (Department of Health 2013a, b, c) and the Keough Review (Department of Health 2013a, b, c).

Nursing care and treatment within inpatient CAMHS settings is poorly defined. Registered nurses in adolescent inpatient settings most often come from a mental health background, and those working in Children's Units may include Registered Sick Children's Nurses (RSCNs). Some inpatient settings also include both learning disability and adult nurses. Unlike in many health specialties this is not the result of strategic workforce design, rather it is the culmination of custom and practice, historical variation in commissioning and attempts to fill vacant posts. This lack of a strategic approach to planning is of concern given that nurses comprise approximately three-quarters of the inpatient CAMHS workforce (NHS Benchmarking Network 2013). As Hadland and Ehresmann (2017) comment, there has been a serious lack of attention paid to workforce development in mental health and more specifically in CAMHS. The Foundation for Professionals in Services to Adolescents (2011) reported that it was common for nurses and care staff who are working directly with young people to have received little or no CAMHS specific training.

It seems unthinkable that a similar such situation could occur in say maternity services or paediatric oncology, which illustrates the lack of parity that children's mental health has when compared to physical health care and provision. Indeed, the Bristol Royal Infirmary inquiry report (Kennedy 2001) recommended that children and young people should always be cared for by health care professionals who hold a recognised qualification in caring for children. It is 15 years since the Royal College of Nursing published a report on the post-registration education and training needs of nurses working with children and young people with mental health problems which included a specific focus on what were identified as the most important training needs for nurses working in CAMHS inpatient settings (RCN 2004). However, no such specialist qualification currently exists for the inpatient CAMHS nurse. The English National Board course number 603, once regarded as the gold standard training for inpatient CAMHS, was decommissioned in the 1990s and there has been no appetite to replace it with a specific nursing award. The adaptation and introduction of IAPT (Increasing Access to Psychological Therapies) into CAMHS inpatient wards is positive, welcome and long overdue. Amongst other skills and competencies, this includes a focus on issues of consent, capacity, confidentiality and the legal framework for children and young people; multidisciplinary assessment and formulation; group processes and team working; and trauma informed care which is fast gathering momentum in mental health care in general.

Perhaps not surprisingly, one of the key challenges facing inpatient CAMHS teams is being able to attract and retain skilled, competent and experienced nursing staff and it is easy to see how this circularity has arisen. There has been concern about the lack of seniority of nurses and the range of therapeutic staff compared to community CAMHS (NHS Benchmarking 2013). In recent years, there has been a gradual workforce shift of nurses from inpatient to community services. This has only added to a challenging situation where the care of children and young people with the most complex and serious difficulties and risks are being cared for and managed by the most inexperienced and poorly prepared staff. In observing this trend, the Quality Network for Inpatient CAMHS (2017) has been concerned about the negative impact on staff morale, team effectiveness and the safety and quality of care. Many stakeholder groups have been concerned about the erosion of skilled inpatient CAMHS nurses in recent years (McDougall 2016). However, this is not a new phenomenon and the gradual decrease in specialist inpatient nursing skills was noted as far back as 1999 as part of the National Inpatient Child and Adolescent Psychiatry (NICAPS) Survey published by the Royal College of Psychiatrists (O'Herlihy et al. 2001).

There has been much debate about the particular skills that inpatient mental health nurses should possess. In 2009, Angela Sergeant (ibid) developed the practitioner's handbook for staff working with child and adolescent. Although this handbook is now 10 years old, the skills and competencies arguably remain current and just as important today. This includes a focus on child and adolescent development, practical interventional skills, risk assessment and self-care for staff. Many aspects of the handbook apply directly to support workers but its use in practice is not widespread. The strategic support of managers is required to release nursing staff to focus on their continuing professional development (CPD), which is now linked to revalidation and recognised as being integral to the overall quality and safety of care (McDougall 2016).

4.5   Summary

As we look back over time, we may conclude that the development of inpatient services for children and young people with mental health problems has not been a strategic process. Rather than being based on evidence of what works and the needs of people who use them, inpatient CAMHS care has evolved and has not always been distinct from residential or custodial care for children and young people.

CAMHS in the UK has its roots in the history of children's welfare services and adult mental health care. There have been many dark periods during this history, and negative aspects of practice intended to rehabilitate delinquent, disruptive or emotionally troubled young people remain in practice in modern CAMHS today. Most notably, these include a culture of restriction and paternalism which is only just starting to transform.

Media reports have been critical of scandals in care but have at the same time called for more beds to be opened for children in crisis. However, inpatient CAMHS admission is not without risk. Whilst hospital admission may be beneficial for some, it can be ineffective or even harmful for others as contagion behaviours associated with self-harm or suicidality can increase. Children and young people who are admitted to CAMHS inpatient units often have backgrounds characterised by high levels of psychosocial adversity. Many have suffered substantial trauma, abuse and loss, which has contributed to their mental health difficulties and risk taking behaviours. They have poor attachments and complex needs, their severe and persistent behaviour problems are difficult to manage in community services and they engage in serious self-harming or suicidal behaviour when faced with perceived threat. Aggressive, threatening or violent behaviour may be placing other people at risk. In this context, it is difficult to see what a time limited inpatient admission can offer beyond physical containment and it is easy to understand why staff may struggle to know what to do to help and resort to control measures, particularly when the necessary staff training and supervision may be lacking.

Inpatient CAMHS wards can be challenging care settings to work in. Supporting children and young people who may use aggression and violence, self-harm or suicidal behaviour to communicate distress, resolve conflict or compete for adult attention is no easy task. Nurses working in inpatient CAMHS must be supported to understand why children or young people behave in particular ways and strive towards enabling a careful balance of authority, responsibility and positive risk taking in helping them to recover. The introduction of trauma informed mental health care is an exciting development and it is vitally important that this is embraced in the CAMHS setting. The education, training and continuing professional development needs of nurses working in CAMHS inpatient care have been neglected during the last 20 years. Most national reviews of CAMHS have highlighted nursing workforce development as a key strategic priority for attention and this is writ large in *Future in Mind*. It remains to be seen if this latest policy brings further clarity to what CAMHS inpatients units are, why they exist and who they are for.

References

Bowers L (2014) Safewards: a new model of conflict and containment on psychiatric wards. J Psychiatr Ment Health Nurs 21(6):499–508. https://doi.org/10.1111/jpm.12129

Bowlby J (1951) Maternal care and mental health. World Health Organisation. WHO, Geneva

Butler-Sloss E (1987) Report of the inquiry into child abuse in Cleveland. HMSO, London

Cameron K (1949) A psychiatric inpatient department for children. J Ment Sci 95:560–566

Care Quality Commission (2012) The essential standards. CQC, London

Care Quality Commission (2017) Review of children and young People's mental health services: phase 1 report. CQC, London

Care Quality Commission (2018) CQC review identifies concerns about the management of child and adolescent mental health inpatient units provided by The Huntercombe Group. https://www.cqc.org.uk/news/releases/cqc-review-identifies-concerns-about-management-camhs-huntercombe

Carr EG, Horner RH, Turnball AP, McLaughlin DM, McAtee ML, Smith CE, Ryan K, Ruef M, Doolabh A, Braddoch D (1999) Positive behaviour support for people with developmental disabilities: a research synthesis. American Association of Mental Retardation, Washington

Cotgrove A (2013) In: McDougall T, Cotgrove A (eds) Specialist mental health care for children and adolescents: hospital, intensive community and home based services. Routledge, London

Cottrell D, Kraam A (2005) Growing up? A history of CAMHS (1987–2005). Child Adolesc Mental Health 10(3):111–117. https://onlinelibrary.wiley.com/doi/abs/10.1111/j.1475-3588.2005.00366.x

Department for Education (2018) Relationships education, relationships and sex education, and health education. https://consult.education.gov.uk/pshe/relationships-education-rse-health-education/

Department of Health (2000) Lost in care: report of the tribunal of inquiry into the abuse of children in care in the former county council areas of Gwynedd and Clwyd since 1974. HMSO, London

Department of Health (2013a) The Cavendish review: review of health care assistants and support workers in NHS and social care. Department of Health, London

Department of Health (2013b) Review into the quality of care and treatment provided by 14 hospital trusts in England. Department of Health, London

Department of Health (2013c) Berwick review into patient safety. Department of Health, London

Department of Health (2014) Closing the gap: priorities for essential change in mental health. HMSO, London

Department of Health (2015) Future in mind: promoting, protecting and improving our children and young people's mental health and wellbeing. HMSO, London

Department of Health and NHS England (2015) Future in mind: promoting, protecting and improving our children and young people's mental health and wellbeing. HMSO, London

Derbyshire Safeguarding Children Board (2018) An assurance report reflecting on the current multi-agency safeguarding arrangements within Derbyshire, with reference to Aston Hall Hospital. https://www.derbyshirescb.org.uk/site-elements/documents/pdf/aston-hall-assurance-report-25-july-2018.pdf

Foundation for Professionals in Services to Adolescents (2011) An analysis of the training needs of frontline staff in inpatient CAMHS. FPSA, London

Francis R (2013) Report of the mid Staffordshire NHS foundation trust public inquiry. Department of Health, London

Frith E (2017) Inpatient provision for children and young people with mental health problems. Education Policy Institute, London

Gingell K (2001) The forgotten children: children admitted to a county asylum between 1854 and 1900. Psychiatr Bull 25(11):432–434

Hadland R, Ehresmann F (2017) Education, training and workforce development for CAMHS nurses. In: McDougall T (ed) Children and young people's mental health: essentials for nurses and other professionals. Routledge, London

Health Advisory Service (1995) Together we stand: the commissioning, role and management of child and adolescent mental health services. NHS Health Advisory Service, London

Hillen T, Szaniecki E (2010) Cyclical demands in demands for out of hours services in child and adolescent psychiatry: implications for service planning. Psychiatrist 34:427–432

Home Affairs Select Committee (2015) Policing and mental health. https://publications.parliament.uk/pa/cm201415/cmselect/cmhaff/202/202.pdf

Horrocks P (1986) Bridges over troubled waters: a report from the NHS advisory service on services for disturbed adolescents. NHS Health Advisory Service, London

House of Commons Health Committee (1997) Child and adolescent mental health services: report, together with the proceedings of the committee. The Stationary Office, London

House of Commons Library (2019) Children and young people's mental health—policy, services, funding and education: briefing paper. House of Commons Library, London

Jacobs B, Green J, Beecham J, Kroll L, et al. (2004) Children and Young Persons Inpatient Evaluation (CHYPIE): a prospective outcome study of inpatient child and adolescent psychiatry in England. In: Presented at the Royal College of Psychiatrists Faculty of Child and Adolescent Psychiatry Annual Residential Conference

Joint Commissioning Panel for Mental Health (2013) Guidance for commissioners of CAMHS. https://www.jcpmh.info/good-services/camhs/

Levy A, Kahan B (1991) The pindown experience and the protection of children: the report of the Staffordshire Child Care Inquiry 1990. Staffordshire County Council, Staffordshire

Masters K (2017) Physical restraint: a historical review and current practice. Psychiatr Ann 47(1):52–55. https://doi.org/10.3928/00485713-20161129-01

McDougall T (2014) Improving quality and safety in inpatient CAMHS. Br J Ment Health Nurs 3(4):148–150. https://doi.org/10.12968/bjmh.2014.3.4.148

McDougall T (2016) Child and adolescent inpatient nursing: a call to action. Br J Ment Health Nurs 5(1):8–12

McDougall T, Nolan TA (2017) Managing behaviours that challenge nurses in CAMHS inpatient settings. In: McDougall T (ed) Children and young people's mental health: essentials for nurses and other professionals. Routledge, London

McDougall T, Worrall-Davies A, Hewson L, Richardosn G, Cotgrove A (2008) Tier 4 child and adolescent mental health services (CAMHS)—inpatient care, day services and alternatives: an overview of tier 4 CAMHS provision in the UK. Child Adolesc Mental Health 13(4):173–180

Mental Health Taskforce (2016) The five year forward view for mental health: a report from the independent Mental Health Taskforce to the NHS in England. https://www.england.nhs.uk/wp-content/uploads/2016/02/Mental-Health-Taskforce-FYFV-final.pdf

Mind (2013) Mental health crisis care—physical restraint in crisis: a report on physical restraint in hospital settings in England. Mind, London

Muir-Cochrane E, O'Kane D, Oster C (2018) Fear and blame in mental health nurses' accounts of restrictive practices: implications for the elimination of seclusion and restraint. Int J Ment Health Nurs 27(5):1511–1521. https://onlinelibrary.wiley.com/doi/full/10.1111/inm.12451

Myers G, Coyle D, Kowalski C, Srinivasan R (2018) How can a young person wait over 90 hours in an emergency department for a bed? Psychiatr Bull 38(5):250

National Audit Office (2018) Improving children and young people's mental health services. NOA, London

NHS Benchmarking Network (2013) CAMHS benchmarking report: december 2013. NBN, London

NHS England (2014) Child and adolescent mental health services (CAMHS) tier 4 report. NHSE, London

NHS England (2018) Child and adolescent mental health services (CAMHS) tier 4: general adolescent services including specialist eating disorder services. NHSE, London

NHS Health Advisory Service (1985) Bridge over troubled waters. HMSO, London

O'Herlihy A, Worrall A, Banerjee S et al (2001) National in-patient child and adolescent psychiatry study (NICAPS). Royal College of Psychiatrists, London

Parry-Jones W (1998) Historical themes. In: Green J, Jacobs B (eds) In-patient child psychiatry: modern practice, research and the future. Routledge, London

Prime Minister's Office (2017). https://www.nhsconfed.org/news/2017/01/prime-minister-unveils-plans-to-transform-mental-healthsupport

Quality Network for Inpatient CAMHS (2017) QNIC annual report. Royal College of Psychiatrists' Research Unit, London

Royal College of Nursing (2004) The post-registration education and training needs of nurses working with children and young people with mental health problems in the UK: a research study conducted by the Mental Health Programme, Royal College of Nursing Institute, in collaboration with the RCN Children and Young People's Mental Health Forum. RCN, London

Sergeant A (2009) Working within child and adolescent inpatient services: a practitioner's handbook. HMSO, London

Smith G, Davis R, Bixler O, Lin H, Altenor A, Altenor R, Hardenstine B, Kopchick G (2005) Pennsylvania state hospital system's seclusion and restraint reduction program. Psychiatr Serv 56:1115–1122

The Bristol Royal Infirmary Inquiry (2001) The report of the public inquiry into children's heart surgery at the Bristol Royal Infirmary 1984–1995

Tulloch S, Lelliott P, Bannister D, Andiappan M, O'Herlihy A, Beecham J, Ayton A (2008) The costs, outcomes and satisfaction for inpatient child and adolescent psychiatric services (COSI-CAPS) study. Report for the National Coordinating Centre for NHS service delivery and Organisation R&D (NCCSDO). HMSO, London

Walk A (1964) The pre history of child psychiatry. Br J Psychiatry 110:754–767

Weiss E (1990) Deadly restraint: a Hartford Courant investigative report. http://articles.courant.com/1998-10-11/news/9810090779_1_mental-health-deaths-restraint-policy

Williams R, Kerfoot M (2005) Child and adolescent mental health services; strategy, planning, delivery, and evaluation. Oxford University Press, Oxford

Wilson C, Rouse L, Rae S, Jones P, Kar Ray M (2015) Restraint reduction in mental healthcare: a systematic review. Cambridgeshire and Peterborough NHS Foundation Trust, Fulbourn

Wolpert M, Harris R, Jones M, Hodges S, Fuggle P, James R, Wiener A, Mckenna C, Law D (2014) THRIVE: the AFC–Tavistock model for CAMHS. CAMHS Evidence-Based Practice Unit, London

Chapter 5
Nursing in Specialist Community CAMHS Settings

Laurence Baldwin

5.1 Nursing in Community CAMHS

In the first chapter, we saw how nurses moved out of their original role in inpatient units when child and adolescent mental health provision developed a more community-based approach. The inclusion of nurses seemed a natural part of a multidisciplinary team, and the fact that nurses were part of those teams seemed to have evolved rather than being a well-planned and thought out part of the development. With the focus on 'New Ways of Working' (DH 2005) and 'Creating Capable Teams Approach' (DH 2007), the focus on skills increased the uncertainty about role definitions and allowed a range of other workers to be part of a multi-professional approach to CAMHS provision. Most recently, in England at least, CYP_IAPT has developed a pathway model of evidence-based care, which relies on staff trained in the particular models of care to deliver the pathways for different conditions. Most NHS Foundation Trusts insist that their staff have an original professional training and registration with a national body, so the main staffing has continued to include staff who are registered with the Nursing and Midwifery Council (NMC), the Health and Care Professions Council (HCPC), or the General Medical Council (GMC). This gives the employers a fall-back position in terms of professional accountability, and ensures a level of assumed competence in basic professional skills for all staff. What it continues to assume rather than define is that these different professional groups have something to offer beyond the ultimate sanction of removal from those professional registers. This chapter then will focus on *how* nurses perform the community CAMHS role more than *what* they do.

L. Baldwin (✉)
School of Nursing, Midwifery and Health, Coventry University, Coventry, Warwickshire, UK
e-mail: ac1273@coventry.ac.uk

© Springer Nature Switzerland AG 2020
L. Baldwin (ed.), *Nursing Skills for Children and Young People's Mental Health*,
https://doi.org/10.1007/978-3-030-18679-1_5

5.2   Nursing Assessments

Prior to the CAMHS Outcome Research Consortium (CORC), there was certainly a lack of standardisation as to assessments, and across the UK individual services varied considerably in how they approached this, usually influenced by the dominant therapeutic model or orientation of the staff involved. In 2002, when I was seconded to the Department of Health for a short while to look at the training needs of staff ahead of the introduction of the National Service Framework for Children (see Baldwin 2005), I had to do a scoping of services in England because at that time they actually did not have a list of what was being provided across England. Generally speaking, the dominant therapeutic model during the 1980s and 1990s was systemic family therapy, so my first community CAMH service was called Child and Family Therapy Services (CAFTS) to reflect this, the term CAMHS itself did not become widespread until after the HAS report (1995) and even then it took a while to be adopted across all services.

Assessments therefore lacked a standardised format in the earlier period of community CAMHS, but would be standardised to a degree within each service, even if there was not an actual form to follow. Clinicians tended to keep a ticklist in their head, which would include family history, developmental history, school and social contextual issues, presenting problem and impact. Risk assessment was not a major issue at this time, and became more important later as services better understood the potential for high-risk behaviour in younger individuals. The dominant culture of family and systemic thinking at the time largely shifted risk issues across to the family as being their responsibility.

One model that did attempt to address all of these issues from a nursing perspective was the 'family nursing' model from Canada (Wright and Leahey 2009), which was first published in 1984 and attempted to marry nursing concepts with the basically structural model of family therapy thinking that was dominant at the time (see Barker 1998). Whilst systemic psychotherapy has since put more emphasis on narrative and postmodern philosophical understandings of human functioning, the structural model has more focus on disruptions to optimal family functioning, the underlying reasons for it, and interventions, which have a systemic impact on changing patterns of family interaction. Wright and Leahey (ibid) saw this as a useful adjunct to a holistic approach to the nursing care of individuals and families, so they brought the two ways of thinking together to create the Calgary Family Assessment and Intervention Model. Their central thinking is that this model is: "... *an organizing framework for conceptualizing the relationship that helps change to occur and healing to begin.*" (p 15) The model is useful in providing some structure, partly based on nursing thinking and partly based on systemic thinking (which places less emphasis on historical factors, and tends to concentrate on the current situation). Nurses undertaking assessments need to consider a range of elements when they conduct an assessment (be it in just one or over several sessions), but also be reflexive enough to understand that their own perceptions and experiences, as well as those of the child, young person and family are inevitably going to shape the assessment and have elements of subjectivity.

Box 5.1 Calgary Family Assessment Model (CFAM): After Wright and Leahey (2009: 52)
Elements of a nursing assessment—CFAM

Structural:
- *Internal*—family composition, genders, sexual orientations, rank order, subsystems, boundaries.
- *External*—extended families, larger systems.
- *Context*—Ethnicity, race, social class, religion and/or spirituality, environment.

Developmental:
- *Stages*
- *Tasks*
- *Attachments*

Functional:
- *Instrumental*—activities of daily living
- *Expressive*—emotional communication, verbal communication, nonverbal communication, circular communication, problem-solving, roles, influence and power, beliefs, alliances and coalitions.

As the model developed and was used in practice, the authors also tried to tease out what nursing skills were being used by family-oriented nurses who employed the assessment and the accompanying Calgary Family Intervention Model (CFIM). The intervention model is essentially structural family therapy based and uses a lot of the tools and techniques of that way of thinking, but Wright and Leahey (ibid) put a lot of emphasis on the employment of nursing skills to effectively employ the model, and the assessment phase, rather than using it as a tick-box exercise. They thought of these in three domains, perceptual, conceptual and executive:

Perceptual skills relate to the ability to make appropriate observations. These are influenced by the individual nurses' own background, experience and training, and are necessarily subjective, but that subjectivity can be mitigated by being reflective on why individuals may interpret what they see in front of them. This domain also includes the ability to observe multiple interactional elements simultaneously within a family in order to inform the thinking about what is being observed and hypothesise on what changes could aid the therapeutic journey.

Conceptual skills involve thinking about what is being involved, and formulating this into a meaningful understanding of patterns of behaviour and interaction. Again there is a degree of subjectivity and the authors refer to 'intuition', although they go on to clarify that actually they are referring to a reflective use of previously learnt skills, which are then consciously brought to bear on understanding the complex situation in practice.

Executive skills are the observable therapeutic interventions which the nurse chooses to make as a result of observing and formulating an idea about what change might be helpful for the family to make.

Whilst these are processes which will be familiar to structural family therapists, what Wright and Leahey do is highlight some of the strengths which nurses have by virtue of their underlying training. Observation skills at a high level are traditionally important for nurses, either physical observations like skin tone, respiration rate and quality, or mental health observations such as mood, responsiveness or heightened reactions. They emphasise the need to engage at a meaningful level that demonstrates care and interest, and the importance of maintaining a therapeutic relationship with different members of the family.

The Calgary Model is useful in illustrating the natural link between nursing's focus on holism and the systemic and social aspects of community nursing. It pulls together and attempts to make explicit the nursing element of a systemic application and gives a framework for a fairly comprehensive assessment and intervention from an autonomous nursing professional (though it also lacks a risk assessment element). As such, it is a good reflection of how nurses in general put their skills into practice prior to the more standardised approach that is required today, though most CAMH nurses were not explicitly using this model. It does, however, assume a level of autonomy which is fast disappearing within current CAMHS practice, and a freedom to spend the amount of time with families that clinical judgement deems necessary, rather than accepting the constrictions that some pathway models assume or dictate. These pressures, and the criticism that the model, whilst comprehensive, is potentially quite time-consuming, led to a 'fifteen-minute assessment' version of the Calgary Model (Martinez et al. 2007), which retained the essential features of the model.

5.3   Nursing Skills in a Structured Assessment Framework

Within a more structured environment, such as that provided by CYP-IAPT, there will be constraints on the nature and style of the initial assessment format. The managerial emphasis may well be on the completion of well-established and formatted assessment tools. As we noted previously the CORC programme, which was voluntary for providers, first introduced routine outcome measures to CAMHS practice (see Hall et al. 2013) and initially used four measures: Goodman's Strengths and Difficulties Questionnaire (SDQs) suite, the Children's Global Assessment Scale (C-GAS), the Health of the Nation Outcome Scale or Children and Adolescents (HoNOSCA), each as baseline and follow up (including discharge) measures, plus the Commission for Health Improvement's Experience of Service Questionnaire (CHI-ESQ) completed at the end of the intervention. Later they added the Goals Based Outcomes (GBOs). Johnston and Gowers (2005) found patchy implementation of these Routine Outcome Measures (ROMs) within CAMHS, but much was learnt from the CORC project prior to the introduction of the broader system of CYP-IAPT, which started in 2011. They took note of this study's findings of a variety of challenges to introduce ROMs, primarily resource-based but also significantly that:

> Another prominent theme was that of concerns relating to philosophical and staff resistance, in that the use of quantitative clinical measures were seen to advocate a psychiatric/medical model, and would be at the expense of qualitative clinical judgements. (Johnston and Gowers 2005: 138)

CYP-IAPT from the start set out to be transformative of services, rather than an add-on to existing services, as CORC had been. It recognised that it must be part of the whole way of treating children, young people and families, unlike the adult version of Improving Access to Psychological Therapies (IAPT), which was aimed at mild to moderate mental health issues and remains entirely separate from other parts of community mental health (Wolpert et al. 2012a). Whilst there was some opposition to the process (Tamimi 2015), and even an offer of an alternative model (Tamimi et al. 2012), the model has been rolled out over several years across England, now covering 100% of the NHS CAMHS provision (Wales, Scotland and Ireland have devolved health administrations) (NHS England 2019). The process has centred on the use of evidence-based practice, in contrast to previous CAMHS practice, which had always suffered from a lack of evidence base and therefore consistency of approach. During the same time period, NICE guidelines had increased their breadth, so more of them included this age range rather than, as previously, focusing on adult mental health. It has also put great emphasis, and continues to do so, on participation of young people, and that is a major achievement which has contributed much to the success of the programme. So this movement has been beneficial in many ways, it has certainly been productive in ensuring that new money came to CAMHS by demonstrating the effectiveness of services, but at a cost of emphasising some elements of practice over others. The programme is largely based on psychological theory, and emphasises the evidence-base of Cognitive Behavioural Therapies (CBT) in particular, though it has been careful to explore the differences in applying CBT theory to young people, which means that more emphasis is put on establishing a relationship with young people and taking longer on this phase than is the case in the more manualised approaches used in adult CBT.

Ironically, the emphasis on participation that has been delivered through the CYP-IAPT programme has not significantly backed up the evidence-base for particular therapies. In an earlier chapter, we looked at what young people want from their therapist, and they largely concentrate on people-based issues, the so-called soft skills that are central to nursing. So while the programme has been uncovering this, it has also pushed for evidence-based pathway approaches to different conditions, because the evidence says that the best way to treat anxiety is with CBT, for example. There is undoubtedly evidence for this, and I would never argue against an evidence-based approach, but what is more difficult for us to provide is the evidence for these 'softer' skills. This is not to say that it is not true, just that it is easier to provide the evidence, in an acceptable positivist way, for some methods of treatment than others, and similarly a positivist approach to demonstrating the value of nursing based interventions will always be more difficult. Most of the mentions of patients valuing certain features of nursing practice that we have looked at so far have come from small scale qualitative studies, and these have a more interpretivist philosophy underlying their methods. By definition, it is almost impossible to generalise the results of these studies because they rely on individual responses. This leaves us with the difficulty of using mostly anecdotal evidence to suggest that the weight of this evidence is cumulative, because the same issues come up in many different areas, yet are hard to bring together as one coherent argument.

Throughout the other chapters, there are examples of outpatient encounters with children and young people, which depend on the quality of the relationship which nurses have been able to develop with young people, and this remains central to the *how* of implementing standardised approaches. Much of the implementation work for the use of standardised assessments has swung to focus on better ways to use the paperwork (or directly inputted answers) in a therapeutic manner (Wolpert et al. 2012b). Allowing the forms to be filled in prior to the first assessment and then giving the clinician more time to pick up the issues raised is one way to do this, but it also means that the clinician needs time to see pre-prepared assessment forms, which can be logistically difficult to arrange, or lead to a pause between arrival at clinic (and collection of the forms, or filling them in whilst in the waiting room) and actually meeting the clinician. This method of working can also lead to awkwardness in raising the issues highlighted in the forms too, if not skilfully handled. Alternatively, the information offered in the forms can interfere with a more natural progression of establishing relationships, and engaging everyone in the room. The information offered on those forms may be partial or lead the clinician to follow one particular line of questioning at the expense of a more holistic understanding of the situation. Some of my most experienced colleagues have fallen into this trap, that of thinking they can see what the primary problem is, and not fully exploring alternatives for what is in front of them. Of course, the biggest mistake that I have heard reported is of getting people to fill in the forms, and then never mentioning them again, in which case you really are getting into the realms of 'feeding the machine' without even trying to use the data.

Box 5.2 The Importance of Language…
Case example:

I usually draw a genogram, or family tree, with families when I first see them. It engages different members of the family, and gives me a visual reference point to refer back to when families are talking about people they are very familiar with, but whose inter-relatedness may be confusing. I used to complete this process by asking 'Is there anyone else in the family who needs to be on this drawing?'

In one meeting with a new family I did this and then, a little further through the session realised they were talking a lot about 'Geoff', who wasn't on the genogram anywhere. I asked who Geoff was, and they told me he was Mum's new partner, who had moved into the home a few months ago, but for some reason was not yet considered 'family'.

After that I started including the question 'Does anyone else live in the house?' which usually elicited lots of information about pets, but did mean I did not miss any significant people any more.

Within the expanded range of forms that CYP-IAPT uses (see their website https://www.corc.uk.net/outcome-experience-measures/), there are a couple of more collaborative tools, which can be used very effectively to co-create therapeutic relationships. Both are mandated for use regularly, and can particularly allow children and young people who struggle with assertiveness to say things they may not otherwise have been able to say unprompted. Goal Based Outcomes (GBOs) we have already mentioned, and they help to put a focus on what is important for the child or young person (although they can also be used to address things that others, parents or even therapists, regard as important to address). These can also be used as part of the discussion about what is working in the therapeutic process, or to look at what hurdles or challenges are currently being faced. Both of these topics can be hard to discuss without a focus for the conversation, so can be used for having difficult conversations about what the young person is experiencing. Likewise, the Session Feedback Questionnaire gives permission for the child or young person to say if they do not feel they were listened to, or if there were things that they did not understand. Clearly, it is important to use this particular scale with a few minutes to spare, rather than at the very end of the session, so that if there are things that need to be addressed the that can be done before time is up. Again, using these forms and not paying attention to the information that you are being given is likely to severely impact the therapeutic relationship—one of the things that we all hate is not feeling listened to. Both these forms then can be used very directly to enhance the relationship and build confidence that the nurse or therapist is actually interested and listening to what is of concern to the individual child or young person. It can also be a way of working out that the child or young person may need different helps to what you are giving, and it is easy to take for granted that we are doing the best thing if we are not checking. Sometimes, we need to admit that we are simply not the best fit for that young person. I once spent many months working with a young woman who was very shy, and I thought she was struggling to verbalise her thoughts and anxieties. Eventually, she got her mum to tell me that she had a phobia about men with beards (which describes me well!) so we had to look for an alternative route forward, and she did much better with a female therapist.

Box 5.3 Making Sure You Are Not Making Assumptions!
Reflective point

One mother I worked with struggled with setting effective boundaries for her two demanding young children, and exhibited a lot of anxiety. We ensured there was good support from the local nursery, and I visited regularly at home to look at how she coped with the high levels of activity her children were exhibiting. I spent time eliciting her thoughts on how she could do things differently, and followed my normal gentle style of being non-directive and empowering.

At a multi-agency meeting, she said that the parenting advice (a directive approach based on simple boundary setting) she had been given at nursery had been very useful, but she was not quite sure if my intervention was much help at all. Actually, she was a bit more blunt than that…

5.4 Risk Assessment and Safety Planning

The issue of risk management (which is not a prominent feature of CYP-IAPT) came into focus in the UK following the Mid-Staffordshire scandal, which led to a lot of soul-searching about how the managerial pressures of the time had led to an atmosphere where compassion and basic nursing practice could apparently be so absent (Trenchard 2013). It also hastened the process of tightening up risk management processes, sometimes more humanely phrased as safety planning, a concept which again fits better with nursing thinking. Within the managerial ethos, however, the response has largely been to introduce standardised risk management systems, which cover the need to document that this aspect of care has been considered and arrangements put in place to respond to crises. This has included the routine and mandatory use of standardised forms such as FACE (2019), or the Beck's Suicide Intent scale (Beck et al. 1979), or increased training for staff such as the STORM training (Gask et al. 2006), or using third sector training such as that offered by PAPYRUS (2019). These mostly focus on suicidal intent as the signifier of level of risk, though FACE (ibid) is a broader scale giving an overall score between 1 and 4 to indicate overall risk of harm and some measure of intensity of input required. Providers tend to use these as a way of demonstrating that they have considered risk, and sometimes to aid clinical supervision, but when they do this it is usually implemented in a bureaucratic manner which mandates, for example, that ALL open cases have an up to date risk assessment, or that everyone who has self-harmed should have a Beck's scale done. This has applicability for those who are at risk, but seems less relevant for a majority of low risk cases. The unfortunate implication of mandating risk assessments for everyone is that it becomes another layer of paperwork (or online inputting), and potentially can just be seen as another 'box-ticking exercise'. If done in a mechanistic style, it can be another obstacle to therapeutic engagement, but for some young people it can be the opposite, a physical demonstration that the nurse (or other clinician) is actively considering the issues around risk, relapse prevention and safety planning. As a Nurse Consultant, I was responsible for introducing this form of standardised risk management into my CAMH service and we took a dual approach to this.

For the low risk cases, the form (we used FACE young people's forms) was always completed after the assessment, and clinical staff were asked to conduct their assessments as normal, allowing therapeutic engagement and the beginning of a therapeutic relationship to develop, but ensuring that during the assessment they covered the areas of the risk management form. After the face-to-face session, the information gathered (in whatever order, as part of the assessment) was filled in across the form and the final score given. Whilst being explicit that this was part of the process, and being considered, clinicians were not expected to have the bright yellow form in front of them during the session and fill each box in, asking the questions for each section in a mechanistic way, and writing them answers down, as a box-ticker might do. Using their own clinical judgement, information was gathered in a more naturalistic way. What this process did was to allow a more natural flow and to use existing skills of engagement, but highlighted to staff that these areas did need covering (in order to complete the form later). It ensured that safety planning was properly considered when it may have been overlooked previously.

For young people with higher levels of risk we involved them much more directly, so thinking about safety planning was much more overt and transparent. Explaining why we needed to think through these issues was much more obvious with young people who were self-harming, for example, and the sections on the form prompted thinking about how aware they were of triggers and relapse dangers, or how they planned to use preventative strategies to try and avoid further episodes. This allowed a much more collaborative and open approach that very actively involved the young people and also clarified that we, as the staff, and the young person were thinking along the same lines and there was no confusion. In some cases, where there was a difference of opinion, it allowed us to explain why we were giving a higher risk rating than the young person would have given themselves, again allowing transparency and openness.

5.5   Case Management and Autonomy

The use of better systems for monitoring caseloads and allowing clinical and management supervision with the community provision of CAMH, but also have arguably diminished the levels of autonomy which was previously the case. Early monitoring of caseload was fairly rudimentary, the original 'Korner stats' approach effectively counted contacts by how many people were in the room (or at the house when a home visit was conducted). This allowed for some fairly creative accounting practices and was certainly not an effective measure of either caseload or workload. My stats as a CPN were always good but then I did a lot of work with large families, so counted each member of the family, which seemed a bit unfair when compared to other team members who did more individual therapeutic work. However, it was also primarily the Community Psychiatric Nurses (CPNs), as we were then, who maintained a flexible approach to engagement and did more of the home visits, which meant that we were out driving around our largely rural area a great deal more rather than seeing consecutive patients in busy clinics, so maybe this evened out overall. It was a fairly unsophisticated approach, as was the piece of paper which was used to monitor how many cases were open to me at any given time. This rudimentary system was also open to abuse in another way, as responding to clinical need often meant that we did not have a mechanism for reviewing regularly how many cases were still open to us, and one audit revealed I had a three figure caseload at one point.

Modern systems can facilitate good clinical supervision and monitor caseload and workload levels, but may restrict the autonomy of clinicians. What was possible in the past, despite the drawbacks outlined above, was the exercise of more clinical judgement in terms of matching pace of progress with individual need. Whilst pathways are good at utilising the evidence-base better, and the children and young person's version of IAPT does recognise this well, there is still an element of proscription in terms of session numbers and review times which may not suit individual pace. The constraints have purpose, they provide more clarity as to goal-based outcomes, for example, and allow a collaborative review of whether those goals have been achieved. On occasion, they can provide a structure which enables this collaborative review to decide to pause interventions, or agree that a mutually agreed ending can be worked towards, and this is in contrast to some cases where endings were difficult to negotiate, or symptoms changed and therapeutic interventions seemed endless. However, the pathways developed under this system usually do have a suggested number of sessions within them, and the temptation is that clinically based decision making and collaborative agreement with children, young people and their families may be over-ridden by managerially driven decisions, particularly in times of scarce resources. This impacts on the clinical autonomy that nurses and others have enjoyed previously, and still manage to retain in some other areas of practice, an autonomy which nurses have typically exercised in the interests of their patients.

5.6   Extended Roles

Elsewhere in this book we have looked at the extended role of Nurse Consultants, which allows quite a high degree of autonomy within a defined sphere of work. CAMHS was an enthusiastic adopter of the role, starting with Marie Armstrong in Nottingham who was the first CAMHS Nurse Consultant, and who remains in post leading the self harm services for young people. Less enthusiastically adopted has been the non-medical prescribing (now independent prescribing) role. This does exist within CAMHS and is most obviously applicable for services such as ADHD clinics where titration of doses and regular medication monitoring is quite labour intensive, and takes up a lot of medical consultant time. As medical consultants have been keen to relinquish some areas of their workload which they consider suitable for others to take over then nurses have taken these roles as an extension of the nursing profile. Outside of prescribing, other areas such as phlebotomy, naso-gastric feeds, and diagnosis or formulation have also been opening up for nurses to step into the space being vacated by doctors. In mental health, the concept of advanced practice has been more difficult to define that in physical health, and arguably the new guidelines, and certainly the available trainings for Advanced Clinical Practitioners (ACPs) (NHS England 2017) seem to favour physical health through the emphasis put on physical clinical examinations. Likewise, the language of multi-professionalism further blurs the difference between nurses and allied health professionals.

Relatively little has been written recently about how nurse prescribers practice differs from that of medical prescribers. Norman et al. (2010) concentrated on the cost-effectiveness of nurses as independent prescribers in mental health (the cost is broadly similar), and the reservations that some service users have, based on the perception that nurses may be less expert than the medical prescribers. The question of whether nurse prescribers performed the role differently, putting more emphasis on nursing skills, so being a 'maxi-nurse' rather than a 'mini-doctor', has also received some attention, though there have been no studies specific to child mental health practice. Cleary et al. (2017) conducted a systematic literature review and found a dozen qualitative studies which have addressed this issue in adult mental health nurse prescribing. Their synthesis of the findings suggested there were strong themes in terms of professional role and professional support, but also that nurse prescribing is generally perceived as more patient-focussed. The study suggested higher levels of consistency in care, and nurse prescribers using their rapport and relationship with service users to enhance holistic care and empower those service users to feel more in control of their medication use. These are important findings, given that service users in other studies have reported difficulties in their relationships with prescribers (see Gale et al. 2012), so establishing and maintaining trusting relationships, a nursing strength, is important both for understanding and developing collaborative approaches to medications within a package of care, and for then agreeing when to change regimes in line with treatment plans. So whilst Noreen Ryan (2007) expressed some caution about the introduction of nurse prescribing into CAMHS she herself did go on to practice as a prescriber within ADHD clinics and described the added value of nurse prescribing (Ryan and McDougall 2009) in terms of timely access to treatment and ensuring that medication is used as part of a wider package of treatment which also includes behavioural advice, school and family support.

Although it is not usually seen as an issue of 'expanded role' there is body of literature on 'nurse-led' services, including some within CAMHS, where nurses have taken responsibility for developing patient-centred forms of service with lower levels of medical involvement and oversight than is traditional, even within multi-disciplinary teams. In mental health the 'nurse-led' element is less fashionable, given the greater overlap of role between professional groups, and the emphasis on multi-professionalism within the workforce literature. Caird et al. (2010) found that nurse-led services in general were both cost-effective and provided significant patient benefits, whilst Castledine (2004) pointed out that this level of autonomy for nurses had some risks, which could be mitigated by effective evaluation activities, and that this kind of service benefits from the transferable skills that nurses bring form other areas of their practice. Not all of these services make an issue of their nature, Marie Armstrong's self-harm service in Nottingham for children and young people has been nurse-led for many years, but does not actively market itself as such. In some cases the nursing culture of just 'getting on', running the services and not making a fuss about the good work we do means we do not get the credit we deserve because of our reluctance to talk about it. Not far from this, the self-harm service in Derby developed from a medically directed service to one run principally by nurses. Again it did not particularly characterise itself as 'nurse-led', but used nursing skills and strengths to transform into a more patient-centred approach (see Baldwin 2013).

Case Example 1: Alli
Alli was 15 when I first met her. She was a prolific self harmer who was referred to community CAMHS following a serious overdose of paracetamol which the liaison team assessed as involving serious intent to end her life. Alli had a strange way of referring to herself, considered herself evil and unworthy of continuing to live, hence her self-destructive urges. She described a constant struggle to maintain a public face which was acceptable to others whilst she was at school or in social situations, and a very different personality when at home. She referred to the public face as 'fake Alli', and the home person as 'real Alli', which led to some questions in people's minds that she might have a psychosis. Initially work centred on keeping her safe and ensuring her parents knew the importance of being aware of her mood and whether she was exhibiting behaviours which indicated a likely further episode of self-harm. The level of support Alli needed in order to feel contained was quite high and for a while she was seen twice a week, eventually dropping to once a week, and for this initial time she continued to self-harm quite prolifically by self-cutting. There was some liaison with school but this proved difficult and Alli spent more and more of her time in the special needs support facilities, finding even this protected

environment difficult and oppressive, and self-harmed even on the school premises.

Sessions focused on trying to understand her thinking, and were quite painful for both of us, including quite a lot of silences whilst we tried to develop some mutual understanding of her pain. As more and more of her thinking became apparent, with marked concrete thinking and rigidity I started to wonder if she might have well hidden autistic traits. I tried to shape her thinking about whether it was OK to be 'different' from other people, rather than seeing herself as evil because she did not fit in the world around her. This met some strong opposition from Alli, who banned me from using the word 'different' for several months... Eventually we managed to look at how some people perceived the world, compared to others, and whether this was acceptable. After a long struggle with this we eventually worked towards getting an assessment and finally a full diagnosis of autism spectrum disorder. This process took over two years, and was a traumatic journey for both Alli and her family, involving some mistaken forks in the road, and ongoing self harm and further suicide attempts. The eventual diagnosis helped Alli to accept herself as having a future, and discover her own way of living which did not involve her having to put on the 'fake Alli' persona in order to survive. Throughout the sessions Alli used poetry as a way to express herself, and I encouraged this as a way of her being able to craft and recraft her words in order to help understand her complex emotions. A local mental health project which used spoken word performance of poetry further helped her with this, and Alli became involved in a community of spoken word artists who were very accepting of her difference. Alli has since published a small volume of her poetry commercially.

My reflections on working with Alli are that a lot of the time all I could do for her was to 'be there' and show her that I was not going to give up on her. Understanding that her way of expressing herself was because she had autism rather than psychosis led to us eventually getting a diagnosis that helped her to understand and accept herself, and finally to stop harming herself. She remains anxious and nervous to this day, but has found her niche and is much happier in herself. In her book she added a dedication that thanked me 'for not giving up on me, even when I'd given up on myself' (book reference withheld to preserve anonymity). Whilst this 'being there' quality of nursing was crucial within the therapeutic relationship that we developed it was not without difficulty within the service. As a Nurse Consultant I managed to maintain considerable autonomy over my practice, but the level and duration of my involvement with this young person was regularly challenged by some within the team as not being in line with practice elsewhere in the service (we were a first wave CYP-IAPT provider). Having enough autonomy to advocate on behalf of the individual needs that Alli had, in order to allow her to access support for long enough to stay safe and develop alternative coping strategies, stretched my nursing convictions and credibility at times, but it proved important in the end.

Case Example 2: Brian

Brian was a 16 year old young man whom I saw at roughly the same time as Alli, and presented very different challenges. I'm using his difficulties to illustrate a much less successful use of nursing skills. Brian presented with persistent low mood which we tried to address initially using some cognitive approaches, in line with NICE guidelines. His mother was a single parent (they had lost contact with his father several years previously), and had struggled with anxiety and severe depression previously. One of her concerns was that Brian was likely to develop an enduring depression similar to her own, and she was keen that he did not suffer in the same way as she has done. Brian had set his heart on becoming a racing driver, and when he suffered damage to one of his eyes which meant he was never going to be able to race professionally he despaired and thought his life was over. The depth of this despair and its fixed nature were unusual, and led to him developing self harming behaviours with some suicidal intent. He became very ingenious in his attempts to self harm, making keeping him safe very difficult, and seriously impacting on his mother's health and left her feeling unable to cope. Brian did not respond well to the SSRI medications we prescribed, and as his depression persisted and his self harming escalated we switched his medication to Mirtazapine, which is not licenced for young people, but seemed to be effective in lessening his low mood symptoms. As the medication became more effective I tried again to engage him with cognitive behavioural approaches to address his thinking, with only limited success, making short bursts of progress only to slip back again each time. Further negative life events lead to further episodes of despair, each accompanied by more self harm and suicidal behaviour. Despite regular sessions over a couple of years Brian was eventually transferred to the care of adult mental health services for ongoing care.

Both Alli and Brian presented risk management or safety planning challenges, and both were at the peak of their self harming behaviours at the same time, meaning I had a very uneasy annual leave over one particular Christmas period, despite putting everything in place that could have been reasonably done. Brian I found much more difficult to engage, he had no way to verbalise his thoughts and feelings, unlike Alli, and I could not find a way to help his mood and feelings of despair. Clinical supervision offered a wide range of suggestions, including the prescribing changes, each of which led to short term improvements, but then a return to the previous state. In many ways I continued with 'being there' and trying every therapeutic option I and my clinical colleagues could muster, but I wasn't able to find the key to help him change. One of the hardest parts of nursing is feeling that you have failed, even if you know logically that you have done all that could be expected, and employed all the skills and experience at your disposal.

5.7   Summary

Do the nursing skills we have talked about here, and elsewhere in the book this match with what children and young want from their nurses and other CAMHS clinicians? In many ways the strengths of nursing, in developing caring therapeutic relationships with them, based on a genuine interest in them as individuals, is very much what we are told they want and need from us. The focus and attention we give to this part of the process seems to be prioritised by nurses because of our underlying training and what we take for granted as important, rather than the more technical aspects of therapies or medications.

What can be difficult, however, is being part of a system which cannot deliver the things that the children and young people we see actually need. Some of them come to understand that, but for many their rage against the system is aimed at us, as the visible face of that system. Over the years my frustration at being unable to deliver the service that I wanted to be able to do was increased by sitting in meetings where waiting list figures were discussed with managers who also cared but had not heard the stories of distress that were read out in the referral meeting each week, so they did not fully see the human picture that each of these figures represented. It would be easy to become complacent, but, whilst we can do the best we can with the children and young people we can see, we must also continue to advocate at a local and national level for increases in service provision.

References

Baldwin L (2005) Multidisciplinary post-registered education needs in child and adolescent mental health services. Nurse Educ Today 25(1):19–22

Baldwin L (2013) Doing the small things right: developing a young person's mental health liaison team. In: Baker C, Shaw C, Biley F (eds) Our encounters with self-harm. PCCS Books, Ross-on-Wye

Barker P (1998) Basic family therapy, 4th edn. Blackwell Science, Oxford

Beck AT, Kovac M, Weissman A (1979) Assessment of suicidal intention: the scale for suicidal ideation. J Consult Clin Psychol 47(2):343–352

Caird J, Rees R, Kavanagh J, Sutcliffe K, Oliver K, Dickson K, Woodman J, Barnett-Page E, Thomas J (2010) The socio-economic value of nursing and midwifery: a rapid systematic review of reviews. EPPI Centre, London

Castledine G (2004) How to run an efficient and safe nurse-led service. Br J Nurs 13(18):3

Cleary M, Kornhaber R, Sayers J, Gray R (2017) Mental health nurse prescribing: a systematic qualitative study. Int J Ment Health Nurs 26:541–553

DH (2005) New ways of working for psychiatrists: enhancing effective, person-centred services through new ways of working in multidisciplinary and multi-agency contexts. Final report "but not the end of the story". Department of Health, London

DH (2007) Creating capable teams approach. Department of Health, London

FACE (2019) FACE CARAS assessment. https://imosphere.co.uk/solutions/face-assessments/toolsets-caras. Accessed 26 Apr 2019

Gale C, Baldwin L, Staples V, Montague J, Waldram D (2012) An exploration of the experience of mental health service users when they decide they would like to change or withdraw from prescribed medications. J Psychiatr Ment Health Nurs 10:853–857

Gask J, Dixon C, Morriss R, Appleby L, Green G (2006) Evaluating STORM skills training for people at risk of suicide. J Adv Nurs 54(6):739–750

Hall C, Moldavsky M, Baldwin L, Marriott M, Newell K, Taylor J, Sayal K, Hollis C (2013) The use of routine outcome measures in two child and adolescent mental health services: a completed audit cycle. BMC Psychiatry 13:270

HAS (1995) Together We Stand: the commissioning, management and role of child and adolescent mental health services. The Health Advisory Service, London

Johnston C, Gowers S (2005) Routine outcome measurement: a survey of UK child and adolescent mental health services. Child Adolesc Mental Health 10(3):133–139

Martinez A, D'Artois D, Rennick JE (2007) Does the 15-minute (or less) family interview influence family nursing practice? J Fam Nurs 13(2):157–178

NHS England (2017) Multi-professional framework for advanced clinical practice. NHS England, London

NHS England (2019) Children and young people's improving access to psychological therapies programme. https://www.england.nhs.uk/mental-health/cyp/iapt/. Accessed 26 Apr 2019

Norman IJ, Coster S, McCrone P, Sibley A, Whittlesea C (2010) A comparison of the clinical effectiveness and costs of mental health supplementary prescribing and independent medical prescribing: a post-test control group study. BMC Health Serv Res 10:4. https://bmchealth-servres.biomedcentral.com/articles/10.1186/1472-6963-10-4. Accessed 26 Apr 2019

PAPYRUS-UK (2019) Applied suicide intervention skills (ASIST) training. https://papyrus-uk.org/applied-suicide-intervention-skills-training-asist/. Accessed 26 Apr 2019

Ryan N (2007) Nurse prescribing and child and adolescent mental health services. Mental Health Pract 10(10):35–37

Ryan N, McDougall T (2009) Nursing children and young people with ADHD. Routledge, London

Tamimi S (2015) Children and young people's improving access to psychological therapies: inspiring innovation or more of the same? BJPsych Bull 39:57–60

Tamimi S, Tetley D, Burgoine W, Walker G (2012) Outcome-oriented child and adolescent mental health services (OO-CAMHS). Clin Child Psychol Psychiatry 18(2):169–184

Trenchard S (2013) Compassion is the key. Nurs Manag 20(5):15

Wolpert M, Fugard AJB, Deighton J, Gorzig A (2012a) Editorial: routine outcomes monitoring as part of children and young people's IAPT (CYP-IAPT)—improving care or unhelpful burden? Child Adolesc Mental Health 17(3):129–130

Wolpert M, Ford T, Trustam E, Law D, Deighton J, Flannery H, Fugard AJB (2012b) Patient-reported outcomes in child and adolescent mental health services (CAMHS): use of idiographic and standardized measures. J Ment Health 21(2):165–173

Wright LM, Leahey M (2009) Nurses and families: a guide to family assessment and intervention, 6th edn. F.A. Davis Company, Philadelphia

Chapter 6
School Nursing and Primary Care: The New Frontline?

Laurence Baldwin and Gemma Robbins

6.1 Policy Context: School Nursing, Primary Care and the Need for Children's Mental Health to Be 'Everybody's Business'

Over the years, and often in the absence of a formalized policy within the UK, nurses have been involved in children and young people's mental health provision within both the school nursing and other primary care settings. This has not been without problems, as we will see, as School Nursing, a specialist area in itself, has primarily been directed at physical health issues within a public health setting, and therefore has traditionally been staffed by registered sick children's nurses with a limited training in mental health (and sometimes a limited interest in the subject too). The growing need to support both school nurses, and also teaching and pastoral staff in schools (both state and private) was identified by Kurtz et al. (1994) in their study of the provision of CAMHS. This led to the idea that a new and specific group of CAMHS staff should offer consultation and supervision, as well as some hands on therapeutic work in the school and primary care setting with children and young people. With the publication of the 'Together We Stand' report (HAS 1995), the role of primary mental health workers (PMHWs) was born (alongside the Four Tier model of service provision), and whilst the PMHW role took a while to develop, it did take off and eventually most areas within the UK had some form of PMHW staffing, acting as a bridge between the frontline of primary healthcare and the more specialist provision of Tier 2 and Tier 3 specialist CAMHS. As time progressed,

L. Baldwin (✉) · G. Robbins
School of Nursing, Midwifery and Health, Coventry University, Coventry, Warwickshire, UK
e-mail: ac1273@coventry.ac.uk; ac4945@coventry.ac.uk

© Springer Nature Switzerland AG 2020
L. Baldwin (ed.), *Nursing Skills for Children and Young People's Mental Health*,
https://doi.org/10.1007/978-3-030-18679-1_6

more questions were asked, mostly by managers who had less understanding of the impact that consultation and supervision could bring, as to why PMHWs were not more actively involved in face-to-face work. The growing influence of metrics in the NHS served to illustrate the number of contacts (face-to-face meetings) that PMHWs were having each week, which generally was less than the contact numbers that their colleagues in specialist CAMHS were achieving. Measuring the impact that PMHWs were achieving in terms of reducing referrals through specialist services, improving public health outcomes, and meeting the elusive goal of providing services at the earliest point of contact to avoid escalation, was far harder to demonstrate. Coupled with the fact that much of the funding for PMHWs had been provided in the rounds of additional public spending following the National Service Framework for Children in 2004 (the first year mandated spending on PMHW or preventative services, and was initially ring-fenced, so had to be spent on this area), the initial glow wore off. Sadly so did the ring-fencing of funds, which had been provided from the Department of Health in England, and that additional funding was absorbed into mainstream social care funding. When austerity hit the country following the banking crisis of 2007/8, and social care departments had to start making drastic cuts in what they were able to provide, the funding for PMHW service was soon lost, though the services struggled on in some isolated areas.

The idea that prevention is better than cure, and an improved general understanding of the mental health needs of children was, however, still being promulgated. The CAMHS Taskforce, set up by the Liberal Democrat Health Minister Norman Lamb, as part of the coalition government, maintained this preventative agenda in the publication of its 'Future In Mind' (2015) policy document. The recommendation within that document was that schools should have a much larger role in identifying and providing care, and that each school should have a mental health champion, in much the same way as they had been required to each have safeguarding leads, and Special Educational Needs Coordinators (SENCOs). What Future In Mind was not able to do, sadly, was to resurrect the concept of PMHWs, so a wide variety of different schemes have developed in the recent past to try and address the needs of Tier 1 provision of mental healthcare for children and young people.[1]

Although additional funding was promised for the implementation of Future In Mind recommendations, there was no ring-fencing of the money given to the commissioning groups, and there is some evidence (Young Minds 2018) that not all of this money did reach the frontline services, some being diverted to other health-spending priorities. Ironically, during this time, the provision of specialist school nursing services has also been under threat, and the pressures on the service make the role extremely difficult to perform (Children's Commissioner 2016).

At the same time, the profile of children and young people's mental healthcare has become more prominent. Whilst Young Minds and the Mental Health Foundation (MHF) had done a tremendous amount of work in the past, it was the adoption of royal patronage of the Place2Be charity that managed to bring more media attention

---

[1] Future in Mind also recommended the end of the four Tier system terminology, hence the use of 'primary care' and 'universal services' phrases within this section of the book.

to the issues, which other third sector organisations, big and small, had been striving to achieve for many years. Whilst the MHF had published the Bright Futures report (1999) describing children's mental health as 'Everybody's Business', and started to promote the idea that children's mental health issues were far more widespread than had been previously recognized; it took a while before other parts of the children's workforce started to think more psychologically and stop thinking that these were just 'CAMHS' problems. The fact that other charities and reports started using the phrase 'everybody's business' to describe their own causes (i.e. King's Fund 2008) showed the success of the concept, but rather diluted the unique message of the report. The readiness of the royal princes (Prince William and Prince Harry) to talk about their own mental health struggles as a result of losing their mother in tragic circumstances whilst they were still children themselves is commendable, and has certainly helped bring the importance of mental health in the younger age group into public focus.

6.2   The Timeline of the School Nurse

School nursing has changed considerably over the years, with the role of the school nurse needing to adapt to the changing environment and needs of children and young people. School nursing originated back in the Victorian era. The specific purpose of the school nurse was to improve children and young people's health, especially those living in poverty and deprived areas. A key element leading to the development of school nursing was a report produced by the British Army (see Wright and Fanning 2014). This exposed the poor health of young men who were joining the army; it was found that between 40 and 60% of army volunteers had been found unfit for service. On further investigation by the government (who set up the Interdepartmental Committee on Physical Deterioration to identify the causes of poor health), it was found that it was not a general health problem, but young men were found to have treatable conditions, which had been left untreated, leading to considerable debilitating illnesses. As a result of this investigation, it was highlighted that not only could the young men not be enlisted in the Army, but also a large number of children were missing a considerable amount of their education due to taking high numbers of sick days. Therefore, it was deemed a matter of urgency to work with children and young people within schools to ensure that their health improved leading to less time away from education (Wright 2011).

This identification of need led to the start of school nursing. As this role began it was agreed that every child and young person should receive at least three medical examinations during their time of education, and clinics were run within schools to treat any health complaints found. It was acknowledged that a main cause of illness was poor nutrition and lack of developmental monitoring to enable problems to be recognised and treated early. Therefore, the main role of the early school nurse was to increase healthy nutrition and monitor the height and weight of children and young people throughout their developmental stages.

This underlying ethos has remained throughout the years, with the key role of the school nurse being to improve health and well-being of children and young people, to reduce the rate of child poverty and to safeguard children and their families. Alongside this, the introduction of vaccinations was established as healthcare progressed. School nurses became the lead in delivering vaccinations to high numbers of children within education. Whilst a number of these roles still resonate today within school nursing, there have also been some significant changes. It can be argued that from the beginning of the school nurse role, there has been a need to acknowledge a child or young person's mental well-being as well as their physical. However, it is evident that this need has increased over the years with what was once a primarily physical care role becoming more and more about the mental and social well-being of our children and young people.

6.3   The Role of a School Nurse Today

School nursing today is viewed as a specialised area of nursing. It is not a standalone role but incorporates a team of nurses at varying levels with different experiences. School nurses make up part of public health teams and all school nurses are expected to engage in further community health study. As a result of this, school nurses today are often referred to as specialist community public health nurses (SCPHN). They work closely with other healthcare professionals such as Health Visitors. Ideally, school nurses should take over the care of children once they reach the age of 5 and start school. The school nurse is then responsible for their health and well-being until they leave school/college at 19. The aim of their role is to ensure that children and young people are given the best possible start in life enabling them to enter adulthood with optimal health.

When considering that the aim of the school nurse is to ensure that young people enter adulthood with optimal health, it highlights the challenge that school nurses face. When you break down their role to analyse the varying care they provide, it includes the following (Public Health England 2018):

- *Health development review*—identifying targeted support that may be required to enable a child to reach their full potential in relation to both health and wellbeing. This should incorporate social care assessment of needs, risks and the choice of the child.
- *Healthy weight*—provide dietary advice and monitor weight for signs of obesity or malnutrition. This should also cover dental health.
- *Targeted support*—identify vulnerable groups and provide specific support for them. Vulnerable groups would include young carers, looked after children, young offenders, asylum seekers, refugees, those living in families where drug use or domestic violence was present, children at risk of abuse or sexual exploitation, and those at risk from female genital mutilation (FGM). Targeted support would also encompass early identification, support and training for complex health needs.

- *Sexual health and contraception*—supporting young people to aid in the reduction of teenage pregnancies and sexually transmitted infections (STIs). This would include providing sessions on puberty, contraception options, pregnancy testing and emergency hormonal contraception.
- *Drugs, alcohol and tobacco*—provide support and prevention of alcohol and drug misuse.
- *Emotional well-being*—Supporting children and young people with their emotional health and well-being. Identifying when intervention and specialised support is required and referring to appropriate services.
- *Safeguarding*—working within the multidisciplinary team to identify and support children and young people who are vulnerable to any type of abuse.
- *Immunisation*—provide immunisations as required and continually reviewing immunisation and vaccine status of children and young people.

It is clear from this role breakdown that school nurses are responsible for covering a wide variety of health and social needs of children and young people at varying developmental stages. When considering the workload, mental health is only a small part of the extensive role. It has taken decades for mental health to be officially recognised within the role and even then, it is discussed in relation to emotional well-being. Mental health and emotional well-being are often used interchangeably; it is important that as healthcare professionals we recognise and acknowledge this, so that we do not misinterpret this as being different from mental healthcare. With this in mind, it is clear that school nurses are facing a significant challenge when identifying mental health distress and providing optimal support and care for a child or young person.

6.4 Challenges Faced by School Nurses When Caring for a Young Person in Mental Distress

It is evident that mental healthcare is not listed or even acknowledged as a predominant role of the school nurse. However, in practice, it is clear that this is a major factor requiring attention. Within the United Kingdom (UK), child and adolescent mental health is a significant public health concern (Membride et al. 2015). School nurses are frontline healthcare professionals often being the first person to engage with a child or young person experiencing mental distress. Working with children and young people to provide support in helping them to cope with the challenges of everyday life is a primary role for the school nurse (Sherwin 2016). Whilst medical advances have reduced the number of infectious diseases and illnesses in children and young people through vaccination programmes, the mental health of our children and young people has deteriorated over the years. It is believed that one in ten school-aged children and young people within the UK will experience a mental health problem (The Children's Society 2014). Therefore, school nurses are viewed as being vital in ensuring that emotional support is provided to children and young people aged between 5 and 19 years aiding in the reduction of potential mental health illnesses or issues developing (Department of Health 2012).

Whilst school nurses are ideally placed to tackle this problem and provide support and care to children and young people in mental distress, there are a number of challenges that they face. School nurses can only address concerns if they are available and present within the school to do this. They are healthcare professionals working within an educational setting with limited medical provision available. They are required to work alongside teachers and support staff, who may have little knowledge of mental health and well-being. The environment within which they can see and assess a child or young person may vary significantly between schools, whilst also being inappropriate for the type of assessment required. This leads to the question, to what extent are these challenges present and how can they be overcome?

6.4.1   Accessibility

Throughout the history of the school nurse role, school nurses have usually been based within education settings. This was greatly advantageous in allowing the nurses to build positive relationships with staff and students. It enabled the nurse to be present whenever students were at school and meant that should a problem arise with a child or young person the nurses were readily available. When considering caring for a child or young person with a mental health illness or presenting in mental distress, it is of utmost importance that they feel comfortable with the healthcare professional and are able to trust them. This type of therapeutic relationship is often not established immediately but can take time and patience. When a school nurse is regularly based within a school, it enables them to build this type of relationship with the students easier, improving the likelihood of a student being able to disclose that they are struggling.

In some UK schools today, you will still find a school nurse based there permanently. However, this tends to only be in specialist schools, where children attending have complex health needs and require regular medical intervention. It is no longer normal practice for a school nurse to be based in one school. Current practice involves having locality teams and nominated leads for areas (Public Health England 2018). The locality teams will include Health Visitors and nurses, who are responsible for caring children and young people within a certain area, covering a number of schools and educational settings. Whilst this does allow a team to be developed, which incorporates a varied skill mix and nurses with differing specialist roles, it can take away the personal element of having one school nurse to cover a specific school. It has been highlighted that children and young people are often reluctant to approach their school nurse due to their lack of interaction with them (Pryjmachuk et al. 2011). Children and young people have expressed a need for school nurses to be more available at times convenient for them and their needs (Bartlett 2015).

Although this may appear like an easily resolved problem by placing school nurses back in schools, the complications around this are great. School nurses would often prefer to be in the schools working alongside teachers and engaging on a daily basis with the students. However, as we can see from the role of the school nurse, they have a very varied and demanding workload. Despite mental health concerns being viewed as high on the agenda, school nurses have to manage this within their given workload (Sherwin 2016). There are key challenges that school nurses have raised in relation to being accessible to children and young people experiencing mental distress. The three predominant ones are child protection (safeguarding children), lack of administrative support and lack of time (Membride et al. 2015). These three factors impact significantly on the availability of school nurses who have to tackle mental health problems. Child protection cases, involving case conferences and numerous meetings, along with the amount of administration work leads to a reduction in time for other activities. A number of school nurses feel if mental health education and support is to be improved within schools, there is a need to consider the provision of mental health advisors (Membride et al. 2015).

6.4.2 Role Clarity and School Provision

Another aspect of the school nurse role that can present as a challenge, when working with distressed children and young people, is their role identification. School nurses are healthcare professionals working with an education environment. The working relationship that the school nurses have with teachers and education staff within schools can vary greatly. Schools differ dramatically in their view and approach to mental health. In one school, teachers could have received training: about mental health illnesses, how to identify a mental health problem and management of illnesses. By comparison, another school may not view this topic as highly and use funding for other activities rather than mental health training for staff. This difference can occur within schools, all based in the same locality and overseen by the same team of school nurses.

When considering these different approaches that schools may take to mental health, it outlines how school nurses will have differing roles within schools. In a school where mental health is viewed with upmost importance, the nurse may be able to provide group sessions, work closely with education staff and actively promote positive mental health and well-being. However, when faced with a school less willing to engage, the opportunities for mental health promotion and awareness will be significantly decreased. It must be acknowledged that one of the problems can often be that teachers and educational staff also have high workloads and are required to prioritise workload in order to meet targets and outcomes. This can often lead to teachers having the same problems as school nurses: there is just not enough time or resources to effectively provide mental health support to children and young people.

Role clarity must also be made clear for students within schools regarding the differing roles of teachers from school nurses. As previously discussed, students often feel that they do not know who the school nurse is or what their role is (Pryjmachuk et al. 2011). For students to feel that they can approach a school nurse, they must understand their role and how it differs from all other staff members at the school. Children and young people can often struggle to see how the school nurse role fits into the educational setting, whilst having concerns that the school nurse will report any appointments back to the teachers. One positive way that school nurses and teachers could work together to improve this is by allowing school nurses to attend assemblies and speak to the students (Pryjmachuk et al. 2011).

As discussed, there are a number of things that can be done to help student awareness around who their school nurse is and what the role of the school nurse entails. However, even if a school is embracing all of these and is promoting the role of the school nurse, there must be an appropriate environment for school nurses to see children and young people. Children and young people in mental distress will often feel vulnerable, isolated and quite scared. Unfortunately, it is evident that a growing number of students are feeling this way due to an acute episode of mental distress or because of a mental health illness (Shapiro 2008). When a child or young person is brave enough to seek help, it is important that the correct environment is available for the school nurse to speak with them and assess them. Ideally, there should be a room in which the school nurse can see a student where they will not get disturbed. When considering best practice, this would be a dedicated room so that students can go there and also access information of support groups, etc.

6.5 Strategies to Aid School Nurses

It is evident that school nurses face a number of challenges when caring for children and young people in mental distress. They have a demanding workload with limited resources and time to meet the needs of the growing number of children and young people requiring support. However, there are a number of strategies and innovative ideas that have positively improved practice within this area across the UK:

6.5.1 Drop in Sessions

Through working with young people and listening to their wishes, drop in sessions have now been established in a number of schools. These sessions will often happen during the students' lunch break and allow students to go to the session and see the school nurse without an appointment. This increases school nurse awareness and allows the school nurse to get to know the students (Sherwin 2016). Although these sessions are not long, they provide vital support for students and positively promote the school nurse's role, whilst providing a safe space for students to discuss any concerns they have.

6.5.2 The Digital Approach

When faced with the challenges of time, resources and the need to provide cost-effective care, school nurses have started to take a digital approach to work with young people (Schuller and Thaker 2015). An instant message service is now being implemented in numerous areas across the UK. An example of this can be found in Doncaster where a team of school nurses set up e-clinics (Schuller and Thaker 2015). These provided an online confidential service for students to access Monday–Friday between the hours of 17.00 and 19.00. This service overcomes some of the previous challenges that have been discussed. It provides students' access to support at a time more convenient for them, and they can do this through their electronic device making it much more accessible than having to physically attend an appointment.

ChatHealth is another digital initiative that has been extremely positive in improving the relationship between school nurses and students. ChatHealth has been designed for young people aged between 11 and 19 years old. It enables them to gain confidential advice from school nurses through a web-based text messaging service. This service is now being rolled out across the UK and recent figures show that one million students have already accessed this service (East Midlands Academic Health Science Network 2018).

6.6 Primary Mental Health Workers: History, Function and Methods of Working

As we noted at the beginning of this chapter, a new role was formed from the Kurtz et al. (ibid) research, which identified the gap between specialist CAMHS and the place where children and young people actually spent a great deal of their time, in school, or in contact with other primary care health services of universal social care services. The outreach function performed by PMHWs relied largely on skills available from specialist nurses, or from specialist children's social workers, so in fact the majority of the PMHW workforce came from these two professional groups, with the addition of some other Allied Health Professionals (AHPs) from disciplines like Occupational Therapy, which also has a mental health focus, and a young person's focus. Most NHS Trusts during this period were keen to mitigate risk in terms of employment by ensuring that they only employed registered healthcare professionals, which meant that these new workers were on relatively high Agenda for Change bandings (usually Band 6, equivalent to a ward sister/charge nurse in an acute setting), and this actually reflected the level of knowledge and experience that they needed. This can be contrasted with current developments, which include the employment of peer support workers, itself a valuable role, but one which does not require a state registered member of staff, and is usually on a lower banding and remuneration. Current efforts to recruit a new range of workers with a year's training but no state registration will also result in a group of staff with no state registration, less experience and a lower banding than the PMHW group that they are destined to replace. Whilst the principle of increasing mental health support in schools is laudable, there are initially only seven trailblazer areas for the Mental Health Support Teams that the government has promised (DfE/DHSC 2018).

Workers in schools whose primary responsibility is for the mental health of the children and young people in that school or primary care setting also need to draw on a range of skills. Traditionally, as we have seen, PMHWs performed less of their role in face-to-face work, and concentrated on enabling school staff to work with young people directly. The rationale for this is largely based on the use of therapeutic relationships, understanding that school staff already have a relationship with the child or young person, which could be used to help them. As we have seen elsewhere in this book, therapeutic relationships take a while to develop, so a face-to-face approach may have some value, allowing the young person to develop a different sort of relationship with a healthcare professional, who is seen as somehow outside of the school system, and this may well be important for some young people who have developed a mistrust of that system, or who have experienced difficult relationships with school staff, which have centred on discipline issues and authoritarian principles. In this case, usually with older young people who have become alienated from the system, then the use of face-to-face work is important, and allows a health or care-based approach as the basis of that relationship. Nurses and others may choose in this case to emphasise their difference from the school system, they may not, for example, be primarily interested in the maintenance of discipline within the school. Whilst retaining an understanding of the need for rules, it is possible to look from a very different angle at the needs of individual young people, based on their pre-existing conditions (such as ADHD or ASD) and become an advocate within that system for creating change for that individual. This 'othering' from the system can be a quite powerful position, though may also need a set of negotiating skills that enable the advocacy to work within the system to create a new understanding of the young person's health needs from an individual perspective. It may create conflict with the system, however, and trying to negotiate for an individual's particular needs within some school systems can be challenging even for experienced nurses who may feel that their own knowledge and experience is not being understood or appreciated by school staff. This reflects very much what the young people themselves may be feeling, and that feeling of frustration with sometimes inflexible school rules and systems can be used to understand the young person's perspective. A degree of personal awareness and reflective skills (as well as access to good clinical supervision) is important when working in these isolated posts, where a lone worker may spend a great deal of time as the only healthcare worker within a system, which has a very different perspective on how that system need to run, and be reacting to very different pressures of targets for attainment.

Being able to explain in clear terms what the needs of individuals and where these come from, in mental health terms, and from a healthcare perspective can be the biggest challenge for school-based staff. The ability to verbalise and articulate conditions, be they neurodevelopmental or based in anxiety or depression, for example, can be a challenge. This becomes a public health task, again one which should be familiar to nurses, of explaining the current understanding of health effects on children and young people. Teachers and other school staff are well-educated professionals, but their education and training has not traditionally included much on the psychology of young people, or their developmental needs. This may be surprising, but generally school teachers in secondary schools have completed degrees in a specialist subject, followed by a year's training in teaching methods, focusing on educational provision and pedagogical technique. Those specializing in primary school teaching may have done a three year degree in teaching of this younger age group which includes some child development training, but again focused on how young people learn, rather than on their psychological needs or how mental health issues affect younger people. Teachers may well be trained in safeguarding children (child protection) and this includes a perspective of sociological understanding, but apart from the school's safeguarding lead this may be limited to a relatively small amount of mandatory training. So whilst some staff undoubtedly have a very good understanding of the psychological lives of their students, many will have a relatively limited grasp of the effects on children and young people of life outside of school, and the attitudes displayed by some staff may reflect the prejudices of the general population. Psychoeducation or public mental health education therefore needs to be ready to challenge the attitudes of some staff who 'don't believe in ADHD' or think that an autism diagnosis is an excuse for poor behaviour. Whilst public awareness has come a long way in the last few years, there remain pockets of very different ways of thinking about mental health within the general population, which may be reflected in school staff and others who provide primary care services.

On a more positive front, there are many teachers and support staff who do develop very good relationships with their students, and these positive supportive relationships can help to get children and young people through difficult parts of their lives. Teaching assistants now have a more formalized training, for example, and often support children with special needs through their school life, usually based on an understanding of the individual needs of young people. In primary and junior schools, where children are largely in class with one teacher for a whole year, this relationship can be fostered to enable young people, and provide them with the support they need. Traditionally, PMHW services would have provided the consultation and supervision to different teaching staff to guide them to understand these relationships and use them in positive ways to support individual need. Again nurses need to be able to understand how these supportive relationships can be used, and concentrate on the skills of empathy and listening, as well as maintaining a positive attitude to encourage the best responses from children. Passing on this skills-based approach within a school or primary care setting can be modelled, but is more likely to be something that needs to be taught in psychoeducational manner, which reflects the core understanding of educational staff. Teaching skills-based approaches, or getting staff to understand that what they may already be doing, based on an intuitive understanding, is actually a skill set in itself, and one that should be valued, is important, again articulating and verbalising the value of apparently simple skills which are often undervalued.

6.7   Third Sector/Charity Involvement

Whilst we have discussed the traditional primary care settings in which nurses work, schooling, both public and private, and elsewhere, NHS and private hospital settings, the landscape is changing and nurses have the opportunity to work elsewhere. The 'third sector' which includes charity and voluntary organisations includes an increasing number of nurse trained staff because the skills and experience that nurses bring are valued as useful. Within these settings, it is important to remember what role you are being asked to do, and how this affects your nursing registration. Childline, for example, is a national phone and online service for distressed children with a clear model of work and includes supervision. Nurses working as volunteers on this, or any other mental health charity, need to be clear as to what advice they are able to offer and use the guidelines of the organization for whom they are acting, rather than falling into a nursing role. At the same time, you would need to be aware that the NMC still considers you to be a nurse, even if you are acting in a different capacity, so some discussion of this potential clash with supervisory staff would be essential to avoid role conflict.

Likewise, working outside of the constraints of the NHS or larger providers means that nurses need to be aware of their vulnerability within an increasingly litigious society. Liability insurance, for example, is something most of us take for granted (it is provided by NHS employers and private providers as part of their responsibilities), but needs to be in place, and should be checked if working for a smaller organization, or if a private practice is established. Rees (2016) has identified some of the advantages of working in an entrepreneurial manner, including the flexibility and agility of smaller consultancy companies to engage in project work or training for a range of providers and commissioners. This level of autonomy can be very appealing or very scary, depending on your outlook.

6.8   Summary

Nurses work in a variety of primary care settings, or in universal care, but this means that they are working with a very different culture, which will have a different dominant culture and outlook. Priorities for the organization in which they are primarily located will not necessarily be healthcare focused, and the need to constantly argue for a different focus can be very wearing. Clinical supervision, and feeling part of the healthcare team is particularly important then you are physically remote from that team and culture for much of the working week. The level of autonomy and responsibility whilst working alone like this can be very freeing, and allows nurses to rely more on their experience and knowledge, but it can also be very isolating.

References

Bartlett H (2015) Can school nurses identify mental health needs early and provide effective advice and support? Br J Sch Nurs 10(3):126–134

Children's Commissioner (2016) Lightning review: school nurses—children's access to school nurses to improve wellbeing and protect them from harm. Office of the Children's Commissioner, London

Department for Education/Department of Health and Social Care (2018) Government response to the consultation on transforming children and young people's mental health provision: a green paper and next steps. DfE/DHSC, London

Department of Health (2012) Getting it right for children, young people and families. Maximising the contribution of the school nursing team: vision and call to action. Department of Health, London

East Midlands Academic Health Science Network (2018) Making an impact. Our work 2013–2018 and our future plans. East Midlands Academic Health Science Network, Nottingham

HAS (1995) Together we stand: the commissioning, role and management of child and adolescent mental health services. The NHS Health Advisory Service, London

King's Fund (2008) Safe births: everybody's business: an independent inquiry into the safety of maternity services in England. King's Fund, London

Kurtz Z, Thornes R, Wolkins S (1994) Services for the mental health of children and young people in England: a national review. Bethlem and Maudsley Hospital, London

Membride H, McFadyen J, Atkinson J (2015) The challenge of meeting children's mental health needs. Br J Sch Nurs 10(1):19–25

Mental Health Foundation (1999) Bright futures: promoting children and young people's mental health. Mental Health Foundation, London

Pryjmachuk S, Graham T, Haddad M, Tylee A (2011) School nurses' perspectives on managing mental health problems in children and young people. J Clin Nurs 21(5):850–859

Public Health England (2018) Best start in life and beyond: improving public health outcomes for children, young people and families guidance to support the commissioning of the healthy child programme 0–19: health visiting and school nursing services. Public Health England, London

Rees D (2016) CAMHS nurses as entrepreneurs. In: McDougall T (ed) Children and young people's mental health: essentials for nurses and other professionals. Routledge, London

Schuller L, Thaker K (2015) Instant messaging: the way to improve access for young people to their school nurse. Community Pract 88(12):34–38

Shapiro S (2008) Addressing self-injury in the school setting. J Sch Nurs 24(3):124–130

Sherwin S (2016) Performing school nursing: narratives of providing support to children and young people. Community Pract 89(4):30–34

The Children's Society (2014) The good childhood report 2014. The Children's Society, York

Wright J (2011) Public health reform and the emergence of school nursing. Br J Sch Nurs 6(6):304–305

Wright J, Fanning A (2014) Transition to the school nursing service. London, The Queen's Nursing Institute

Young Minds (2018) Children's mental health funding not going where it should be. https://youngminds.org.uk/about-us/media-centre/press-releases/children-s-mental-health-funding-not-going-where-it-should-be/. Accessed 26 Apr 2019

Chapter 7
Paediatric Wards and Children's Emergency Departments: Wrong Place or Right Place for Seeing Distressed Young People?

Gemma Robbins and Stephanie Mansfield

7.1 Introduction

High numbers of children and young people attend Emergency Department's (ED) within the United Kingdom every year requiring treatment, care and support for a mental health illness. A large percentage of these will be admitted to children's wards for further care. Historically, the number of children and young people attending ED and requiring hospital admission in mental distress has been minimal. Over the last 10 years, there has been a significant increase in ED attendance along with hospital admissions. Therefore, children's nurses are required to enhance their knowledge whilst utilising their existing skills in order to provide optimal care for this patient group.

Whilst all fields of nurses will share a particular skill set, there are clear differences in practice between the nursing specialisms, which must be acknowledged and recognised. Kraemer (2010) highlights how a medical/surgical patient will follow a linear route of care, for example, tests are carried out, a diagnosis is formed, and a treatment plan created. However, a patient in mental distress will require a circular route of care in which no test can clearly offer a diagnosis and treatment plan. These different routes of care can be reflected in nurses' skills and practice. A children's nurse will often be very task-orientated knowing exactly what is required to treat and improve a patient's symptoms. However, a mental health nurse is much more likely to understand the importance of taking time to sit with a patient providing a safe space for them to express how they feel. A mental health nurse will view spending time with a patient as a therapeutic intervention, in the same way a children's nurse provides therapeutic care through the administration of drugs and physical interventions.

G. Robbins (✉)
Children and Young People's Nursing, Coventry University, Coventry, Warwickshire, UK
e-mail: ac4945@coventry.ac.uk

S. Mansfield
School of Nursing, Midwifery and Health, Coventry University, Coventry, Warwickshire, UK

© Springer Nature Switzerland AG 2020
L. Baldwin (ed.), *Nursing Skills for Children and Young People's Mental Health*,
https://doi.org/10.1007/978-3-030-18679-1_7

When considering these differences, it is evident that nurses from varying fields will bring different skills and knowledge to patient care. Thus, highlighting the challenges children's nurses face when caring for children and young people who are presenting in mental distress. This chapter will explore this in detail, discussing how children's nurses can apply their current skills to practice. We will also address the environmental challenges of healthcare settings when caring for a child or young person in mental distress.

7.2   Current Guidelines

A key question that appears to be central to the start of this chapter is: why are children and young people with mental distress assessed in ED and admitted to general children's wards? This has been an ongoing debate and central discussion point between healthcare professionals for a number of years.

Whilst the Royal College of Paediatrics and Child Health (2018) outline that community mental health services should be working with children and young people prior to them reaching crisis point, it is recognised that due to underfunding, time restrictions and waiting lists of such services, this cannot always be achieved. Thus, children and young people in mental distress often seek support at a point of crisis within emergency care services. Evidently, some children and young people will require physical care to counteract drug overdoses or assess and treat injuries. Therefore, it is essential they present to ED ensuring these physical needs are cared for alongside supporting their mental health. The ED as stated within its name is for emergencies; therefore a person suffering mental distress should be seen and treated with the same concern and priority as those with physical emergency needs.

The National Institute of Clinical Excellence (NICE) guidelines (2004; 2011) clearly state that all children and young people should be admitted to a children's ward for assessment and care prior to being transferred to any specialist unit. Whilst service delivery varies between areas, in general there are no specific units for the initial assessment and care of a child or young person in mental distress. Child and adolescent mental health services (CAMHS) provide specialised units that admit patients who require a higher level of mental health care and more intense treatment. It has been recognised that if a child or young person were to be admitted to one of these areas for initial assessment and treatment it could have negative implications for them, and inadvertently cause greater distress. Hence, the guidelines outline that children's wards are the optimal place for children and young people experiencing an acute episode of mental distress.

Whilst a high number of children and young people are admitted to hospital due to experiencing differing levels of mental distress, only a small percentage of these patients will require further care within specialist inpatient areas. The majority of patients can be safely discharged back into the community and receive the care they require outside of specialist mental health inpatient facilities. Children's inpatient wards provide a pit stop of care to identify patients' mental health needs, deescalate crisis point and ensure planned therapy and follow up are in place for the child and family.

With this in mind, we must acknowledge that although a large number of patients being admitted with a mental health complaint are acutely unwell, there will be cases where you encounter a child or young person who is seriously unwell and requires specialist services. A key skill is to be able to identify the difference between the acutely unwell patient and the patient who has a serious mental health illness. However, as we will discuss in detail later in this chapter, the overarching factor is how do you care for this patient group and what skills are transferrable between all patients experiencing mental distress?

Box 7.1 Time Out
- Before continuing this chapter, take a moment to think about the different symptoms you have seen in ED and on the ward area.
- What were the predominant care needs of this patient group and what skills did you utilise when caring for them?

7.3 Patient Presentation

You have spent time thinking about different symptoms and how a child or young person presents when they are in mental distress. From completing this exercise, you have probably noticed that children and young people in mental distress will all present differently. In order to understand the skills required to care for this patient group we first must establish the key difference between caring for a medical/surgical patient and a mental health patient. For the majority of patients you will already know: how a patient will present dependent upon their diagnosis, exactly what to prepare and what tests are likely to be required. This is not the case for a child or young person in mental distress. Whilst some patients may present frustrated, loud and uncooperative, another patient may be quiet, withdrawn and accommodating to your requests. One patient in mental distress may not be at risk of self-harm or suicidal behaviour whilst another may be high risk and require one to one care.

So how do we as children's nurses distinguish this? Taking time to talk to our patient. Patients will not all present in obvious mental distress, they may attend an ED with an unexplained injury, a mechanism of injury which does not seem appropriate or abdominal pain to which no obvious medical/surgical cause can be obtained. Thus, children's nurses are required to use their skills to detect symptoms or subtle changes in patients. Whilst we follow a structured ABCDE approach to assessment for all patients, nurses should also use their senses to assist in identifying patient symptoms. A patient suffering mental anxiety should not be treated any differently.

Picture a patient you have cared for with mental distress. Imagine they have again presented to you in practice. Use the categories to think about your assessment.

7.3.1 Sight: What Do You See?

- Obvious physical injury—burns, cuts, bruising etc. Does this appear to be a previous injury (scars) or is this more recent in appearance.
- Where can you see?—Patient clothing? Is this appropriate for the time of year— could they be trying to hide themselves. Sinking back into their clothing etc.— could this be due to the environment—consider noise/sensory overload.
- Appearance—Does the person look unkempt, have pride in their appearance, trying to hide certain aspects, signs of vomiting? Do they look pale, clammy, and unwell?
- Behaviour—How is the child or young person acting? Introvert, Extravert. Does this change? When? Why?
- Relationship—who is the patient accompanied by? Does the patient appear comfortable with this person? Does their demeanour change with differing people?

7.3.2 Smell: What Do You Smell?

- Does the patient have any medical conditions? Diabetes (pear drop), Wound infection and sepsis. Medical conditions should always be considered initially alongside a patient's mental distress especially in patients who appear confused. Diabetic ketoacidosis and sepsis can present with confused patients displaying combative behaviour.
- Alcohol, illicit drug use and legal highs—the majority of patients will not have ingested alcohol or used any illicit drugs. However, some may have done so to try and combat their feelings or in an attempt to enhance their feelings. Use of alcohol and drugs such as cannabis may be detected through their strong smell. However, patients should always be asked regardless as differing substances can elevate feelings and change behaviours.

7.3.3 Taste: Here Think About the Patient, Possibility of Ingestion and the Effects of the Patients' Feelings on Their Intake

- Ingestion—Talk to the patient and carer. Ask if the patient has ingested anything—medications, illicit drugs, alcohol, and objects. If so when, how much? How did they feel at the time? How do they feel now?
- Patient intake—Again ask the patient and carer. Are they eating, drinking? How much? When? Does their mood affect this?

7.3.4   Touch: What Did You Feel?

- Observations—A full set of observations should be taken for patients on attendance to ED. Taking a manual pulse also enables detection of pulse rhythm and volume. Does the patient feel clammy? Skin turgor—does the patient appear at risk of dehydration—is this fitting with alleged intake?
- Obvious wounds—Ask the patient first to examine any wounds. When did these occur? Does the patients account fit with the wound? Signs of infection? Has the wound been cared for? How? Document size, appearance, actions taken.

7.3.5   Hear: What Can You Hear?

- Listen to the patient—What are they saying? Are they saying anything? How are they speaking—confidently, quietly? Is someone else speaking for them—is this at the child's request or are they not being allowed to speak?
- Difficult questions—Difficult questions will need to be asked dependent upon the situation. Did you wish to harm yourself? Do you want to harm yourself now? Do you have plans to harm yourself? Do you feel suicidal now? Do you still wish to take your own life? Do you have plans to take your own life now?

Listening to children and young people during times of mental distress is often what children's nurses find the most difficult. Whilst nurses pride themselves on their communication skills and ability to communicate with children of differing developmental ages, it is often asking difficult questions and listening to these answers which nurses find uneasy. Some professionals can become scared by silences or by asking such direct questions. However, it is essential these questions are asked to establish how the child or young person was and is feeling and talking to them to establish what therapeutic techniques they may wish to engage in to deescalate or distract themselves.

It is important that as nurses we can reflect not only on our practice, but how a patient can alter our feelings and highlight our fears. Research has shown that as children's nurses we are very task orientated and often feel most rewarded in our work when we are able to complete our set tasks. This becomes much more difficult when caring for a patient who does not require tasks, but rather our time and assistance in easing their psychological pain. We cannot ease this by administering pain relief or offering drug therapy. Research suggests that when a nurse is unable to ease the pain and improve the symptoms, they are left feeling inadequate and like they have somehow failed the patient (Menzies-Lyth 1960). If we are to move forward in identifying our skills and how we can improve the care delivered to children and young people in mental distress, we first must acknowledge what our own struggles and fears are when caring for this patient group.

Box 7.2 Time Out
- Write down your concerns/fears of caring for children and young people with mental distress?
- Having thought about your patient, did you consider the elements in each category?
- Would you adapt your practice now to assist in your assessment of a patient?
- During the rest of the chapter think about what you have already done in practice to combat these concerns and what you will do differently from now on.

7.4 Factors to Consider

When considering whether children's wards and ED are the right or wrong place for this patient group, a number of factors must be considered. Research would suggest that children's nurses have a good understanding of mental health symptoms, illnesses and problems. However, this knowledge alone is clearly not enough to enable a children's nurse to feel confident in caring for this patient group (Fisher and Foster 2016). It is evident that children's nurses feel that a number of challenges can cause barriers to providing optimal care for this patient group. Children's nurses face the problem of time, environment, mental health knowledge and the unknown. All of these play a part in creating a barrier to ensuring that children and young people in mental distress receive optimal care and provision when attending the ED and being admitted to a children's ward.

As we work through this chapter, we will break down these barriers. Although, we can clearly see that these would provide an argument for why ED and wards are not the right place for this patient group, we will also examine how some of these challenges can be overcome by incorporating current and new skills into everyday practice.

7.5 Time

Time is a key challenge when caring for this patient group. If you were to observe the nurses' journey through their shift, you would see that this is a constant challenge that must be overcome for optimal care to be delivered to the child or young person in mental distress.

This issue of time can start before the nurse has even met their patient, in ED and ward hand-over; some patients in mental distress are often viewed as "light" patients who require little input. After all they are just waiting to be seen by the CAMHS team. This is the first point at which time factors can be addressed and altered. If a child or young person in mental distress were to be viewed as requiring time with as much importance as a child requiring intravenous antibiotic therapy, then at the very start of the shift patient allocation would allow the nurse time to talk, understand and listen to their patient.

The ED also has added pressures of triage, patient flow and waiting targets. Patients presenting should have an initial assessment within 15 min of arrival. This ensures patient safety is maintained (The Royal College of Emergency Medicine 2017). Initial assessment of those presenting in mental distress must consider not only physical observations but the mental capacity and psychological pain the person is experiencing. A child or young person who requires immediate physical care for a wound or overdose will clearly take priority in triage category. However, those who may not be suicidal but are experiencing crisis point in other ways may not be so obvious in their need for immediate attention. As discussed previously, all patients present differently which can sometimes be difficult for nurses to establish the severity of a person's distress. Children's nurses have the skills to detect subtle changes and communicate well with children, young people and families but may feel unsure when triaging certain patients. A tool such as the Australian mental health triage tool (Australian Government Department of Health 2013) can be adapted for children and young people and used as a guide for nurses to use when considering the prioritisation of patients being seen in ED. Nurses should also ensure documentation of questions asked to patients, especially those outlining if a patient has been or still is suicidal or self-harming.

This patient group may also present the issue of patient flow. The ED relies on patients being able to move through the department either to a point of discharge or admission. In order to enable patients to continue being assessed and treated it is essential patients have a plan for definitive care. Patients experiencing mental distress may not all require admission however this is the decision of the CAMHS team in conjunction with ED medical and nursing staff. Social care services may also be involved and therefore must be consulted. Therefore, patients may be required to stay within ED for longer than the four hour waiting time target. Many hospitals will have interim observation areas, taking the patient 'off the clock' but enabling them to stay longer in hospital without admission. However, this is not always available and dependant on the demands of the CAMH service can sometimes lead to long waits for a plan of care to be established. Thus meaning children, young people and their families are caught in an uncertain middle ground unsure of a definitive plan of care. ED services are also placed in grey territory as observation areas are only to be used as an interim gateway and patients should not be placed here to save admission or the four hour target. If children and young people are then waiting lengthy amounts of time for CAMHS assessment (dependent upon the demands of the CAMH service) this places added pressure on ED from perspectives of patient flow and ensuring quality patient care. Ultimately each situation is different and ED coordinators will always consider the needs of the patient and family first when assessing the options of a patient's journey.

If differing services are involved, such as social care, this will impact on time to discharge as all services must be happy the patient is safe to return into the community. Whilst all healthcare professionals involved should document conversations with differing services within a child's notes, sometimes these can be difficult to distinguish between entries and cause a repeat of conversations with services and ultimately a delay in discharge. A separate call log sheet can be useful in patient's notes which can be used throughout their patient journey to log calls made to services such as CAMHS and social care (Birmingham Children's Hospital 2016) (see Example 1 at end of chapter). The log clearly documents the conversation held, time, name and contact of the professionals spoken to allowing easy access to information and phone contacts if required.

Another delay may be due to finding an appropriate ward area for the child or young person to be admitted to. Consideration is required to ensure not only the safety of the patient but also other inpatients already on the ward. Patients may need to be moved within the ward and staffing reconsidered to maintain and provide a good standard of care to all patients. We discuss this in more detail further in the chapter.

The challenges discussed highlight a further issue of building trust with the patient. As stated previously nurses have the ability to communicate with a wide range of people in ever-changing situations. However, in ED especially, patients will be in contact with many differing healthcare professionals and enabling a consistent person to be with the child or young person throughout their journey can be difficult. Depending on the running of the area, some patients may see at least three nurses prior to being admitted to the ward area (Triage, majors nurse and observation area). This does not account for possible shift changes or break cover. Therefore, trying to build a trusting relationship in a short space of time with a patient who is suffering mental distress can be challenging. Patients need stability and time to bond with their nurse, to build a relationship where they feel comfortable to speak, answer questions and not feel anxious of continuous changes of professionals. For this reason, time is needed to be spent with this patient group to establish these foundations and staff consistency must be maintained wherever possible.

This leads to the next area of time that must be overcome, the view that talking to a patient and/or playing a game with them is completely irresponsible when the clinical area is busy. When a child or young person presents in mental distress then they must be given time to talk and express how they feel. It is important that as healthcare professionals we remember that psychological pain can be just as debilitating as physical pain. Although we cannot give pain relief in the same way, offering a channel for a child or young person's psychological pain can be extremely beneficial. This can be done in a number of ways:

- Play a game
- Sitting enabling a safe space for the child or young person to talk
- Art
- Offering pen and paper for the child or young person to write how they feel

It can be useful to view this as a form of therapy; rather than offering pharmacological therapy you are offering alternative forms of therapy which are the most effective for this patient group.

Another consideration is to allow time in your day to sit with the child or young person for 5 min. It is apparent that this can be difficult as not all children and young people will want to talk, and it can often feel uncomfortable when a child or young person will not engage with you. However, it is important to remember that often a child or young person may not be able to articulate how they are feeling. It may be the first time they have felt this way and they do not understand it themselves, making it nearly impossible for them to then explain it to a healthcare professional. Another consideration is their developmental age and life experience. For example, if a person has never lost anyone then they will not know what bereavement feels like. Children and young people are often experiencing emotions like anger, betrayal or bereavement for the first time. You will often find that your presence alone can have a positive impact, reiterating to the child or young person that they do matter, they are worthy of your time and that you do care. You may even find that taking five minutes twice a day to sit with them will lead to them attempting to share with you what is happening and what their struggles are.

In the bustling climate of ED spending time to sit with a patient may seem impossible. Nurses must consider their patient load and prioritise time to attend the cubicle to sit with their patient suffering mental distress. Whilst undertaking observations, there is an opportunity for nurses to not only check the physical aspects of the child or young person's health, but also to sit and talk with the patient understanding their mental health needs. If a patient does not require frequent physical observations then nurses should not see this as time saved for a differing patient task but endeavour to set themselves this time as the opportunity to speak with their patient in mental distress, gauge how they are feeling and if there are any further therapeutic techniques they could implement. Making positive small changes to practice can enhance patient care.

Whilst it may appear that the above discussion does not require any specific skills, it is actually quite the opposite. As nurses we are taught throughout our nurse training and career that communication skills are vital, and of upmost importance in delivering high quality patient care. In order to communicate effectively with a child or young person in mental distress we need to master the skill of silence. Many people can become uncomfortable when sitting in silence or when there are quiet pauses in conversation. However, for a child or young person struggling with mental distress the chance to process their thoughts and how they feel is important. If there are no silent opportunities for this to happen the likelihood of them being able to share their feelings is reduced.

Another time concept that is worth considering is the way a child or young person is feeling when they are experiencing an episode of mental distress. It is possible that their self-esteem is quite low, they are feeling frightened due to being in a new environment and they do not know who they can trust. When healthcare professionals factor time into their day to sit with this patient group it can help alleviate all these factors. It enables the child or young person to feel that they are important, it gives an opportunity for them to ask questions and understand how things work in the clinical setting and reinforces that the nurses and staff are there to help and support them.

7.6   Environment

Environment is a long-standing concern for nurses caring for children and young people in mental distress. If you were to enter a CAMHS unit you would certainly notice significant differences from a general children's ward. Child centred EDs and children's wards are environments providing a child friendly setting with age appropriate décor, games, toys and activities. However, they are also areas full of clinical equipment and clinical procedure areas. You will find at every bedside a number of clinical elements such as oxygen and suction. You are not likely to find such a clinical setting in a CAMHS unit. In these settings it is more common to see lounges, open spaces and rooms that would resemble more of a "home from home" style bed space.

This difference in environment can provide a challenge for healthcare professionals. A key factor in nursing practice is ensuring that the patient is safe at all times (Nursing and Midwifery Council (NMC) 2018). Whilst the clinical equipment and environment provides a required level of safety for the majority of patients, it inadvertently acts as a hazard and concern for children and young people at risk of engaging in self-harm/suicidal behaviour. The most common reason for a child or young person who is mentally unwell being admitted is due to them engaging in a form of self-harm/suicidal behaviour. This leads to the predominant priority being to keep the child or young person safe from further harm.

This challenge is managed through the utilisation of assessment and prioritisation skills. Dependent upon the level of risk of further self-harm/suicidal behaviour then it would be expected that a bed space near the nurse's station would be allocated to allow for close observation. It would also be necessary to clear the bed space of hazardous items such as oxygen and suction tubing.

In the ED allocation of a cubicle or bed space may not be so obvious due to the differing floorplans of each setting. Time should be taken to consider the most appropriate cubicles for patients in mental distress, nurses are then aware of which areas are safer for patients who may be at risk of self-harm/suicidal behaviour. Ideally cubicles should have two entrances for patients who may present with an aggressive nature, as staff safety must also be considered. Equipment should be able to be removed including all wires and tubing not only from the bed space but the trolley itself. Gloves, alcohol gel, etc. should also be removed for risk of ingestion. If clinical equipment is required for a physical need then this should be minimal, dependent upon the patient's circumstance and be re-evaluated as a patient's condition changes. Nurses should document the removal or changes made to the cubicle and reasoning why. At this point, nurses should also consider the patients belongings. Whilst children's nurses do not have the authority to search patients or their belongings they can request patients show them the contents of bags, etc. and ask if patients have any objects, tablets, drugs etc. they could use to harm themselves with. This may appear invasive to ask such questions however, it is essential to maintain the safety of the child or young person and others in ED or the ward environment. This is not to say the patient with mental distress may harm others but more of concern is another patient potentially picking up a bag containing a blade for example and injuring themselves. Evidently, the patient may not tell the truth as they fear repercussions if they do have a substance or object with them. This is where building a trusting relationship is essential. As discussed before children and young people need to feel they can trust the professionals caring for them in order to feel able to speak out and provide honest answers. Nurses must ensure the patient is aware that they may need to inform other services if necessary and remove any risky items. However, they will be with the patient to support them throughout and be able to assist in working with them to find alternative ways to overcome possible anxiety of not having a blade with them, as an example.

Even when all the best efforts are made, ED and wards areas are full of equipment and hazards that cannot be removed or avoided. With this in mind, the nursing ratio level must be addressed in order to optimise safety for this patient group. Patients in mental distress will require close observation and monitoring. When considering nursing ratios, it must be acknowledged that there are currently no clear ratio's available to guide nurses in their practice. It is expected that the nurse in charge will assess this regularly in relation to patient needs and level of care required. This highlights that maintaining safety is a challenge when children and young people in mental distress are cared for within ED and children's ward settings.

This may appear to be a negative view of the ED and ward environment and the implications this has for both healthcare professionals working within these areas and children and young people in mental distress. However, there is no alternative option for this patient group as no other units, assessment methods or wards exist that will cater purely for their needs. With this in mind, we must consider the positives of this environment and what skills healthcare professionals can bring to not only enhance the clinical environment but also reduce the hazard risk for this patient group.

From our experience of working within these areas, we have found that it is common for close monitoring and observations to consist of viewing the patient from a distance and completing paperwork to state whether they are awake, what they are doing and whether there are any signs of concerning behaviour. Whilst this is less time consuming than engaging in conservation, allows the patient the privacy of not being disturbed, ensures that they are still where they should be and they are displaying no apparent signs of distress, it does not highlight the actual psychological state of the child or young person. This is the key piece of information that will provide guidance on whether this child or young person is likely to attempt or successfully engage in further self-harm/suicidal behaviour. As healthcare professionals we should never be afraid to ask the question of how are you feeling? Do you feel anxious? On a scale of 1–10 (with 10 being 'Very' and one 'Not at all') Do you feel the need to self-harm? This openly asks the question of how they are feeling, allows identification of anxiety and the need to self-harm to be acknowledged prior to it worsening. If this can be identified, then often things can be put in place to aid the reduction of the child or young persons' anxiety before it escalates.

For healthcare professionals who are new to this type of assessment and care, try to equate it to managing physical pain. In the same way you would use a scale to monitor physical pain and ask the patient how they feel, you can transfer this skill to assess psychological pain with a patient in mental distress. Mental distress can be simply defined as psychological pain, a very real pain but one which cannot be numbed with analgesia. With this in mind, you can then consider asking the child or young person questions like:

- How anxious are you feeling?
- How busy does your brain feel?
- How tense and stressed are you feeling?

All of these questions can be used incorporating the same 0–10 scale that you would use to assess physical pain.

Similarly, consider the environment around the child or young person at the time, how is this impacting on the mental distress of the patient. Children and young people who present to hospital with autism or other learning disabilities should have their individual needs catered for with regards to preferences/dislikes. For example, if a child becomes distressed in busy, noisy areas they should be taken to a quieter area which they feel comfortable within. This also applies to the patient in mental distress. Picture yourself in a new environment feeling anxious, nervous and confused about how you are feeling, having lots people around you whom you do not know, it is noisy, people talking, crying, machines beeping. This would be overwhelming normally but even more so when patients are already feeling distressed and vulnerable. This overload of senses may be too much for some children, so assess the situation and endeavour to ensure the child is in a more suitable environment for them at that time. Again, this can be difficult especially in a bustling ED but nurses should work with the child or young person and their families to ensure the best possible outcome is achieved.

7.7   Mental Health Knowledge

A key concern which would strongly advocate for children's wards and ED being the wrong place for this patient group is the knowledge and understanding staff have in relation to mental health. When students decide they want to be a nurse, from the start they need to choose which field of nursing they would like to go into. Children's nursing and mental health nursing are two separate nursing specialisms. This immediately seems to cause a divide between exactly which patients' nurses' care for and what skills each field possesses.

Despite this clear divide, it is important to look at the skills each nurse brings, rather than the skills they may not have. Whilst a children's nurse has not studied mental health illnesses, symptoms and treatment plans in depth they still have a vast array of skills that benefit this patient group. A children's nurse learns quite quickly the importance of communication and how this needs to alter significantly dependent upon the developmental age of the patient. This is a transferrable skill that can be used with any patient irrespective of their diagnosis or illness. Patients presenting in mental distress often require a gentle approach and an understanding that they may not be able to articulate how they are feeling. A sensitive approach to communication, taking the time to ensure the patient feels comfortable and safe, enhances the possibility of the child or young person opening up about how they are feeling and what is going on for them. This high level of communication is a transferrable skill that children's nurses can offer.

Children's nurses are also skilled at identifying a deteriorating patient based on both physical and behaviour cues as well as clinical observations. In the same way, a child with a respiratory complaint may become breathless, quieter, pale, etc. when entering respiratory distress; a young person in mental distress may become breathless, quiet and pale should their anxiety increase to a level at which they have an anxiety or panic attack. This skill of observation and being able to identify presentation changes in a patient is a transferrable skill, it can be used with patients experiencing physical or psychological problems. Although an in-depth understanding of different mental health illnesses may not be present, a children's nurse still has skills that greatly benefit children and young people in mental distress. The identification changes of physiological and psychological changes allow for interventions to be incorporated into care in order to improve patient outcomes.

These skills need to continue to be nurtured and enhanced dependent upon a nurse's area of care. Whilst training in many areas focuses on more physical-based skills, it is essential to recognise that nurses require continued development of skills in caring for patients in mental distress. Likewise, clinical supervision also needs to be considered. Children and young people presenting with mental distress may display all differing behaviours. They may have differing levels of wounds or physical care needs and may disclose very sensitive information to nursing staff. Similarly to child protection cases where staff require supervision to assist in reflection and talk through upsetting cases, nurses coming into contact with patients suffering psychological pain should have time to discuss and reflect on their actions. This could also assist professionals to detect any reoccurring issues with processes followed, work to ensure patients are receiving the upmost care and staff feel comfortable and confident in caring for this patient group.

7.8   Summary

It is evident that answering the question of whether wards and ED are the right or wrong place for distressed children and young people is by no means simple. Whilst it is clear that children's nurses within these areas do offer a range of skills, knowledge and experience to care for this patient group, they face a number of extenuating challenges that do not present with all other patient groups. Overall, there a number of positive and negative elements as outlined below:

Right Place:

- Allows children and young people to be assessed and initially cared for in a general children's environment as oppose to a specialist unit which may heighten their distress.
- Children's nurses have exceptional communication skills that can be adopted and incorporated to provide a safe place for children and young people to express themselves.
- Children's ED and children's wards provide an environment which has been designed with children and young people in mind.
- Children's ED and ward areas have healthcare professionals who are trained in distraction techniques along with offering a number of games and activities providing temporary distraction from the current problem.

Wrong Place:

- Children's ED and wards are designed to keep children with physical ailments safe, therefore, not providing optimal safety for a child or young person in mental distress.
- Children's ED and ward areas are busy places with uncontrolled levels of activity and noise which could heighten levels of anxiety for already distressed patients.
- Staff ratios do not incorporate or consider the level of supervision and care a child or young person in mental distress may require.
- Staff knowledge in mental health care can be limited dependent upon their experience and the training that has been made available to them.

So, what can we do as children's nurses to ensure our patients are cared for effectively? Think about your area of nursing and current practices for children and young people in mental distress.

- Could more time be made to spend with children and young people and how could this be done?
- Could the environment be adapted?
- Do staff require more training?
- If so, could a designated nurse with interest in mental health disseminate knowledge from training courses to other staff?
- Is supervision in place?
- If not, could this be put in action?

Small changes in areas can make a big impact in improving patient care and staff confidence. Whilst the debate will continue, and opinions will be divided as to whether ED and children's wards are the right or wrong place for this patient group, we as children's nurses can ensure more tailored care is achieved.

Example 1: Services Liaison Form

Patient Name   Sam Smith   Hospital number   A12345678

Date and time	Team contacted/ contact no and person spoken to E.G. ERA, social care	Comments (conversation held)	Practitioner name Print and sign
22nd March 2019 08.20	CAMHS crisis team Alan Jones— 07123-456789	I have informed Nurse Alan Jones of Sam's reasons for attendance to ED today. I have informed him that Sam is with mum, currently settled and has been assessed and treated for minor self-harm wounds to her wrist. Medically she is fit for discharge however she requires a CAMHS assessment. Alan reports staff are currently finishing morning handover and a member of the team will be attending the hospital to assess Sam shortly afterwards. Whilst an exact time cannot be given as there are other patients also awaiting assessment in hospital, CAMHS will attend ED when they arrive to provide an updated estimated time of assessment.	Stephanie Mansfield RNC
22nd March 2019 08.50	Social care Sally Mills—0123 456 6789	I have informed Sally Mills from children's social care of Sam's reasons for attendance to ED. Sally will inform Sam's social worker this morning. Nurses are to contact Sam's social worker again once CAMHS have assessed her to inform social care of Sam's care plan and ensure follow up care is arranged.	Stephanie Mansfield RNC

References

Australian Government Department of Health (2013) Mental health triage tool. [online] Available from http://www.health.gov.au/internet/publications/publishing.nsf/Content/triageqrg~triageqrg-mh. Accessed 2 April 2019

Birmingham Children's Hospital (2016) CAMHS liaison pack. Birmingham Children's Hospital, Birmingham

Fisher G, Foster C (2016) Examining the needs of paediatric nurses caring for children and young people presenting with self-harm/suicidal behaviour on general paediatric wards: findings from a small-scale study. Child Care Pract 22(3):309–322

Kraemer S (2010) Liaison and cooperation between paediatrics and mental health. Paediatr Child Health 20(8):382–387

Menzies-Lyth I (1960) Social systems as a defence against anxiety. An empirical study of the nursing service of a general hospital. Hum Relat 13:95–121

National Institute for Health and Clinical Excellence (2004) Self-harm, the short-term physical and psychological management and secondary prevention of self-harm in primary and secondary care. National Institute for Clinical Excellence, London

National Institute for Health and Clinical Excellence (2011) Self-harm: longer-term management. National Institute for Clinical Excellence, Manchester

Nursing and Midwifery Council (NMC) (2018) The code: professional standards for practice and behaviour for nurses, midwives and nursing associates. Nursing and Midwifery Council, London

Royal College of Paediatrics and Child Health (2018) Facing the future: standards for children in emergency care settings. The Royal College of Paediatrics and Child Health, London

The Royal College of Emergency Medicine (2017) Initial assessment of emergency department patients. The Royal College of Emergency Medicine, London

Chapter 8
Helping Children and Young People with Eating Problems and Disorders

Katrina Singhatey and Moira Goodman

8.1 Introduction

The desire to feed others is primal. It is one of the most important ways we can show we care. It is also an incredibly important part of daily life. Whether taking others for lunch or dinner, celebrating birthdays and special holidays, giving sweets and chocolates as gifts, food surrounds us. We do not just eat and feed others because of hunger, food provides pleasure. Eating food, preparing food, cooking food, even growing food, all have social dimensions. Within different faiths, food also marks important events, Christmas, Hanukkah, New Year, Eid, Divali, Valentine's Day, Easter, Mother's Day, or Father's Day, and many others, every celebration seems to include food.

But food is also essential to our survival. At its most basic, without proper nutrition, we get ill and die. When we have children, our first instinct is to feed them. When we feed our children, it makes us happy and fulfilled. If food is scarce, it is common for parents to feed their children over themselves. When food is in abundance, parents are likely to indulge their children with their favourite foods. It is the most basic way of nurturing another being.

When we begin to notice our child is not eating as they should, we question why. Babies may be lactose intolerant, unable to digest particular foods, or unable to tolerate particular textures, fussy eaters could have neurodevelopmental difficulties. As parents, we take note of likes and dislikes and can be alert to changes in eating habits. So, whilst losing appetite could be a sign of a physical illness, or a virus, or intense sadness rather than a problem with eating itself, we are aware that over eating can also be a sign of a physiological problem. Changes in eating can invoke a

K. Singhatey (✉)
Cognitive Behavioural Psychotherapist (Private Practice), Nottingham, UK

M. Goodman
Retired, formerly Nottinghamshire Healthcare NHS Foundation Trust, Nottingham, UK

© Springer Nature Switzerland AG 2020
L. Baldwin (ed.), *Nursing Skills for Children and Young People's Mental Health*,
https://doi.org/10.1007/978-3-030-18679-1_8

powerful emotional response in parents and they can often seek help to determine what is wrong.

For parents too there can also be a sense of social shame when a child is not eating as we think they should. We are judged if our child is too thin or too fat, too fussy or perceived as greedy. We want to be seen as good parents, so if we feel judged by others, it can also have a profound effect on how we feel as parents. Complicating the matter is the way in which this may be differently perceived in different cultures, and parents will employ various strategies in order to get the child to eat what they believe to be the correct diet. Parents may first ask for advice from immediate family, grandparents, friends, neighbours, then Health Visitors, doctors and other professionals in attempts to address the eating problems in their child.

It is so important to be aware of the differing emotions in parents and how long they have been battling with these feelings when they come to us for help. It is also vital to understand that the child or young person may have been experiencing internal and external angst for quite some time too. Therefore, the family that you see in front of you initially, when they are at crisis point, will most likely not be an accurate reflection of how they were prior to the difficulties they are currently experiencing.

8.2   A Skills-Based Approach to Assessment

This chapter is the only one which looks at a single issue, rather than taking a broader view of applying skills, and it will do that by looking at a series of case studies as a way of demonstrating HOW skills are applied in this difficult treatment setting, as well as highlighting the process used to apply those skills, which draw from a range of different theoretical approaches, but apply the techniques using what we have seen to be nursing approaches. Although this chapter concentrates on eating disorders, it does not set out the very important guidelines used in the formal treatment of anorexia, bulimia and other eating problems. Other books have done that well (McDougall et al. 2017) and it is particularly important that nurses and others are aware of the importance of physical healthcare alongside psychological care in the treatment of eating problems, which have the highest mortality rate amongst children and young people's mental health issues (Smink et al. 2012). NICE guidelines in the UK (NICE 2017), for example, set out the latest thinking on treating these issues, and the well-regarded MARSIPAN (RCPsych 2014) document is also vital. Recently, in the UK additional funding has focused on the Maudsley guidelines (Eisler et al. 2016) as a framework for treatment within the English specialist services, which have received additional funding and training. All of these documents will tell you WHAT to do, we are concentrating on HOW to make these strategies and guidelines effective by using nursing skills to engage children, young people and families.

The guidelines quoted above all stress the need for assessors to undertake the task of assessing thoroughly, sensitively and with compassion. Because of the many possible reasons for eating difficulties and disorders, a detailed developmental assessment is usually necessary. Assessors should use and encourage curiosity in family members during this process. We need to explain exactly why the assessment is essential in getting to understand the experience of the entire family and that during the process young people and their carers may discover some lovely things about themselves and how others see them. We also need to let them know that at any time, if they disagree with what someone else has said, they can interrupt and provide their version. This is so everyone feels that their opinion is valued and that they are respected in the process, but may not be something that families are used to doing. Systemic and family therapies stress the need for curiosity to be used in this way to gently elicit information in an acceptable manner rather than using a more formal developmental history taking approach, which can appear to be a box-ticking exercise (i.e. DAWBA 2012). Likewise, it is important that an assessment is structured to gather information without being too overwhelming (Wright and Leahey 2013).

The initial assessment should provide lots of information. When asking parents about their own individual backgrounds, if there is genuine curiosity then supplementary questions, about how they met for example, can be taken positively and more information may be offered, often to the delight of the young person, who may not have heard these stories, and start to see their parents in a new light. However, if the parents are feeling particularly judged and appear suspicious, then it is best to avoid pursuing this angle, even if it is deemed important, until you have gained their trust. Questions about early development can be made fun. Rather than sticking to a simple set of questions about developmental milestones, you can ask what the young person was like as a very young child, what they liked and disliked, who their friends were, how they separated from their parents at nursery and school. These questions can more gently uncover any early signs of developmental delay, separation anxiety, personalities and childhood relationship difficulties.

Whether parents remain together or live separately and how this is managed is useful information. The nature of relationships with step-parents, half or step-siblings are also crucial to making sense of how the family functions. If the child or young person is adopted or fostered, then there may be less detailed information to work with. As long as we can glean as much as we can in a carefully considered manner which inspires trust and a sense of coming together for the same aim, that is the most important aspect in developing the basis of a therapeutic relationship. Whilst this is being done in a manner which aims to develop a therapeutic rapport, we may be told something that is worrying to us. Unless this requires immediate attention, such as hospitalisation or the removal of the young person to prevent imminent harm (under safeguarding or child protection rules), everything should be noted and any concerns should be voiced openly and options or ways forward discussed together with the family and young person respectfully.

Sometimes, following assessment, it becomes fairly clear what has happened and how it has happened. It is essential that we present this hypothesis to the young person and the family to see if it fits with their understanding of the difficulties. It may be that we have missed information, which leads us to rethink our ideas and come up with a new hypothesis, so checking is important, rather than assuming we know what is going on, a common failing with 'experts'! If our ideas are validated then planning a way forward with everyone's consent is of the utmost importance. Care plans can then be formulated together and further appointments made. Letting the family know exactly what they should expect of the service is not only good practice, but it also reminds the young person and family that they are not alone and will receive the support they require.

Communication with the GP is essential and another key component of any care plan. We are always going to be part of a wider healthcare (and often social care) team, so clear communication about who is performing what role within the team is essential. Practitioners need to know that checks and tests have ruled out physical health causes and routine blood tests may be necessary because restricted diets can deprive the body of important nutrients, and bingeing and purging can interfere with the balance of electrolytes in the body. Assuming that someone else is doing this can have tragic consequences, so make sure that communication is good, and let the young person and family know that you are talking with other parts of the wider team.

With younger children, it is possible that sadness, bereavement, bullying and insecurities within the family have precipitated the eating problems. It makes sense therefore to address these difficulties with the family and the social systems that surround them. A parent becoming unemployed, money being tight, or welfare benefits being withdrawn can also cause a sensitive child to react to the tension in the home by reducing their food intake. Parental mental or physical ill-health can also cause stress and pressure within the home and lessen the appetites of young people through stress and worry, which is why in-depth thorough assessments can be vital. These are sensitive issues, which need to be approached through an angle that is empathic and non-judgmental.

Sometimes, what begins as an eating problem can turn quite quickly into a disorder. Once the initial assessment has been completed, it is important to remember that all assessments are ongoing and with each subsequent session, more information may come to light as the family and young person feels safer and more able to trust the practitioners. Some sessions may be undertaken with the young person by themselves or just with the parents or caregivers.

8.3 Anorexia Nervosa

There are many theories about anorexia nervosa—remember that 'anorexia' on its own can be used to describe not eating for other reasons, the 'nervosa' describes the psychological element. The commonly accepted medical model tends to focus on identifying potential causes, and, depending on assessment outcomes, developing treatment plans to address those causes and any subsequent effects accordingly. Theories of aetiology, the potential causes, range from 'flawed' parenting, family mental health, bereavement, an overly strict, rigid or pressured home environment, childhood trauma or abuse (see Rikani et al. 2013). Clinicians, under this model, are encouraged to explore environmental reasons for the anorexia, which can lead very quickly and unwittingly into parents and carers feeling blamed for the illness in the child. This has the potential to cause further rifts in family relationships and can in itself hinder treatment and damage already fragile relationships.

We know that many parents and carers of young people who develop anorexia are high achievers (Halse et al. 2007). Many are perfectionists, middle class, often in high profile jobs. Do they put pressure on the young people in their care or do the young people feel that they have to live up to what they perceive to be parental expectations, or are they actually just very much like their parents, with a similarly driven personality themselves? To avoid this trap of blaming either parents or child, which can lead to a very negative reaction and disengagement from therapy, relationships need to be explored in depth. Whilst the guidelines we have talked about discuss the importance of a family history and understanding of family interactions, it is important to be clear with the parents or carers, and with the child and young person why so much emphasis is being put on this aspect. The medical model of finding a cause and then treating it is very familiar to anyone who has had contact with healthcare professionals, it is the dominant way of thinking, but no-one likes to think that THEY are the cause of someone else's distress or illness. In working with young people and their families, parents may therefore blame themselves or each other, consciously or subconsciously, and they will be searching for answers, wondering what they have done wrong. Because of this dominant way of thinking about illness, they are likely to be believing that if they can put their finger on the trigger, then they can help to make their child better. Any added inference of blame by professionals will therefore only add to their sense of shame.

The young person can, and often does, also feel guilt. They may feel guilty for putting their parents through emotional turmoil whilst also feeling driven to continue along their path because no one understands what they are going through. They can become secretive, hiding their eating habits and weight loss from those around them and also hiding their thoughts, feelings and fears. Ironically, this often compounds the problem, so when the extent of weight loss is discovered the parents feel even more guilty for not having noticed.

By the time young people are referred to specialist mental health services, parents have already realised there is a problem that they feel helpless to solve. They can feel confused and frustrated. They may well be asking themselves why is this happening to my child? Why won't my child eat their favourite foods anymore? Why are they throwing their lunch away? Why are they now insistent on eliminating certain foods from their diet? Why has my carefree child turned into a silent stranger? Often, young people cannot answer their parents' questions. They can be just as confused about what is happening to them as everyone else. They do not understand either, yet feel compelled to continue on their path regardless. Getting a young person who is experiencing this for the first time to explain themselves to a stranger when they cannot even explain it to themselves is incredibly difficult.

This is why we felt that in order to provide the best service possible to the young people and families that we were working with, we really needed to find a better way to understand what this particular set of young people were going through. What had distorted their thinking patterns so much and sent them on a path of self-destruction? In our search for understanding, we came across a book written by Peggy Claude-Pierre: 'The Secret Language of Eating Disorders' (1997), which gave us new insights to so many of our questions. Peggy, a parent herself and a psychologist, had begun to notice the signs that other parents had spoken about, in her eldest daughter. These manifested in changes in mood, changes in behaviour, changes in eating patterns, making up excuses not to eat with the family, becoming withdrawn and secretive and hiding her weight loss under baggy clothes. As a parent, she took her daughter to see specialists, where a diagnosis of anorexia nervosa was made.

In her book, Peggy wrote about feeling blamed for her daughter's illness. She described the intensive assessments and evaluations by professionals searching for a cause and the impact that had on her entire being as a parent. The main conclusion of the professionals was that other than refeeding, there was little else that could be done. Her daughter was described was manipulative by some healthcare professionals, whilst others assumed there had been sexual abuse in her earlier years and another group said it was a fear of growing up into a young woman that was the cause. Peggy knew her daughter well. She knew that she was unusually sensitive to, and aware of others' needs, and attended to them diligently. She wrote about her determination as a parent not to give up. She described her need, as a psychologist herself, to really understand what had happened to her daughter and find a way to help her. It was Peggy's close relationship with her daughter that not only enabled her to ask, with genuine curiosity, what she was thinking and feeling? It was the love and trust between them that allowed her daughter to answer openly and honestly. Her daughter told her that there seemed to be a voice in her head that was much louder than her own and even though she knew it made no logical sense, she felt compelled to obey it. The fact that her daughter had always been very logical confused Peggy and they began to explore these alternative thoughts together. One day, whilst driving in the car together, her daughter told her: "... you see these traffic lights? I know they are on green but my head is telling me that for me, they are on red. It is as though I am not allowed to go through even though others can." (ibid page 13).

Over this period of time, Peggy found that it was the distorted thoughts that were fuelling the anorexia. Her once confident daughter had begun to doubt everything. She had became so indecisive she could no longer make everyday small decisions and needed enormous amounts of reassurance. They discussed this loud voice in her daughters head which Peggy named 'Confirmed Negative Condition' (CNC). In a joint attempt to separate CNC from her daughter, they began to explore everything the voice was saying. Her daughter was then able to use her mother's strength as her own by sharing exactly what the voice was saying to her when it was saying it. It was a punishing voice, an insulting voice which questioned everything she did. Nothing was right. The voice became louder and more punitive. In order to eat even small amounts of food which she knew, logically, could not sustain her, she was forced to negotiate by agreeing to exercise or skip another meal. The voice also told her she was unlovable, ugly, fat and stupid. This voice was unrelenting but by agreeing to join forces with her mother, she was able to allow a more gentle and compassionate voice to slowly begin to fight the CNC.

We read about this journey towards recovery and through it we gained some insight into the minds of those suffering with anorexia, the answers to many of our questions and a compassionate and respectful way to work with and to successfully treat this disorder. We were inspired by the fact that not only did Peggy successfully treat her daughter, she then went on to set up her own clinic and residential home for those who had battled the disorder in vain for years yet were able to recover under her care. The people she treated described these unrelenting voices in their heads, voices telling them they were undeserving, unworthy of a place in this world, unlovable and despicable, the voice generated self-hatred in them. They truly believed that death through starvation was the only course left for them. Peggy's book gave us so much insight into the mind of anorexia, it provided us with the tools we felt we needed to fine tune our treatment approach.

The CNCs that Peggy referred to were already well known to us through other ways of conceptualising them, as 'internal voices', or negative automatic thoughts (NATS) which are well described in the Cognitive Behavioural Therapy literature (i.e. Kinsella and Garland 2008). Importantly, Peggy's book does not describe the 'voice of anorexia', as we came to think of it, as being an external voice, which is more characteristic of psychosis. NATS are already well understood as a driver in depression and a maintainer in Obsessive Compulsive Disorders (OCD). In these circumstances, our usual self-chastising internal voice becomes louder, more punitive and self-deprecating in depression, or more and more demanding in OCD. This causes us to believe what it is telling us regardless of how illogical it may appear to the outside observer. We decided to call this 'the voice of anorexia' because it serves to distance the voice inside the mind from the behaviour of the sufferer. Peggy used the negative thinking versus the positive thinking technique called externalisation in systemic psychotherapy (Boston 2000) which distances the behaviours and compulsion from blame. She described feeding the positive and starving the negative as a powerful treatment tool.

We realised that we had to keep in mind the description of how all of the assessments made Peggy feel and how she described parents feeling tortured by the misplaced belief that they are the cause of their child's condition (ibid page 7). We decided that above all, we would centre our assessments around curiosity, adopt a non-blaming stance with understanding and would respond sensitively with compassion, gentleness and respect. The following case examples will describe in some detail how we were then able to enact this approach to developing therapeutic relationships with the children, young people and families, and (usually) use this approach to facilitate their recovery.

Case Example One: Annie

The first young person who was referred to us following our exploration of anorexic thinking and the impact this illness has on all family members was Annie aged 11 years old. An only child, she attended the first appointment with her mother and father. We explained the assessment process to them and said we would try to make it less boring than it sounded. Annie was pre-pubescent and in her final year of junior school, and both parents were educated middle class professionals. Annie was a meticulous child, very obedient, studious and serious. She preferred not to speak much in that first session but instead opted for her mother to speak on her behalf. We reassured her that this would be fine but just asked her to speak out if her mother got anything wrong. All her developmental milestones had been reached and in fact Annie had been quite advanced in many milestones, crawling, walking, language development and fine motor skills were all acquired earlier than usual. Annie's mother was a teacher and had taken time off to spend the first few years of Annie's life at home with her. Her father travelled frequently for business so her mother undertook the majority of the parenting.

Our technique of allowing the mother to speak on Annie's behalf, with the understanding that Annie would interrupt if mother got some things wrong, worked well. Annie began to interrupt her mother more and more often, and as she felt more confident to communicate with us, she divulged more information. She had delighted at hearing how she was as a baby and toddler, and when her mother talked of Annie's struggles separating at nursery, Annie said it was because she preferred being with her mummy to being with strangers and other small children. We then asked each family member to tell us about a special memory they had of Annie growing up. Annie talked about a wonderful holiday they had taken together. Mother and father joined in, providing their own memories of that particular holiday a couple of years beforehand. They laughed together and when we asked what was their favourite food memory, each gave us different accounts while they enjoyed remembering together. We explored other current aspects of daily living. There was no bullying, and Annie maintained close friendships with her peer group. There had been no family bereavements, and Annie had close relationships with grandparents on both sides. She was doing well at school and seeing friends outside of school. Annie had always been a fussy eater but when we broached the subject of eating, we were met with initial silence from Annie and both her parents, in contrast to their previous discussion of less difficult matters. As a way of overcoming this sudden silence we asked if it was OK to read out the referral letter from the GP, and told them we needed them to let us know if the GP had got anything wrong.

The GP's referral letter indicated that mother had become concerned because her fussy child had become more and more fussy over the past few months. Annie had begun to restrict her diet and no longer wanted to eat what had used to be her favourite foods in the evenings and at weekends. Her portions became smaller and smaller and she was visibly losing weight. Mother had phoned school and she discovered Annie had begun to throw her lunches away. Annie was clearly embarrassed by this and had retreated back into her uncommunicative self. She had sunk back into her chair and looked smaller somehow. We gently explained why we needed food to eat and that we were there to help her get back to how she used to be. We related this back to how they had told us she had been on the holiday. Her mother then talked about this happy go lucky child who loved to do so much with her had become withdrawn and had lost her sparkle and how she had been wondering whether Annie was becoming depressed. Annie's father, who had said very little up to this point, suddenly spoke up. He said there was 'an elephant in the room' that no one was talking about. We asked him what he meant and he said that Annie's mother had been bulimic for years so it was not surprising to him that this had caused Annie to develop her own eating disorder.

The atmosphere in the room changed again. Annie's mother seemed compelled to discuss her own relationship with food and how she would eat normally with everyone else for a month or 2 followed by a month where she survived purely on slimming shakes in order to stay within a particular weight range. She looked visibly deflated and it seemed that the blame and guilt in the room were both very powerful emotions. We could see from Annie's face that she had heard this many times before and she herself felt guilty for hearing her mother being blamed. We suggested that it would be a really good idea if we saw the parents alone for the next session because it seemed they had things to discuss that were not necessarily directly linked to the difficulties their daughter was experiencing but could possibly have an impact on her treatment.

Both parents welcomed the opportunity to talk about this particular issue and Annie seemed pleased and relieved that they were going to do so. We asked permission to weigh her so we could get an accurate view of her struggles. Her Body Mass Index (BMI) was 15.[1] We then asked Annie if she felt able to complete a food diary over the next fortnight so we could see what she was eating. We also asked her to note how easy or difficult it was for her at each meal and reassured her that our aim was to help her get back to the young person she was on the holiday that she remembered so fondly. And prior to organising further appointments, we asked each one individually how the experience of that first appointment had been for them. This may seem like a minor aspect of the first appointment but in doing so we are reinforcing our commitment to the family. It reminds each family member that we are listening and are respecting and valuing each voice.

Relating this back to our new way of thinking we reflected that we could have heard the words 'bulimic mother' and decided that we had found the cause and gone down the route of suggesting mother get her own help. Instead, we decided to acknowledge that mother was bulimic, acknowledge that there were parental rifts because of this and the connection to their daughters eating difficulties and to acknowledge that this was affecting their daughter's emotional wellbeing. We decided more information was needed and parents would benefit from a discussion without the presence of their daughter.

Seeing the parents together was enlightening. Father initially presented as very angry and blaming. Mother talked about her guilt and began to cry, and then her husband, upon seeing this, softened in what he was saying. He had not realised how much she had been silently blaming herself. We took the time to discuss with both parents what we knew about eating disorders and bulimia, particularly the common

---

[1] Whilst BMI is not a perfect indicator of difficulties, particularly in younger children, we have used it throughout this chapter as a rough guide to where different individuals lay in comparison to the 'average' BMI of 18.5–25.

need for control because the fear of being out of control was so strong. We talked about the belief that many bulimic people have that if their weight is not controlled, then nothing can be controlled and the result will be catastrophic. Father was both shocked and saddened that his wife had been going through this alone. She, in turn, said she felt so relieved that others could understand the emotions she was dealing with. We then went on to explain that although there are many theories about why someone begins to restrict their diet, a bulimic mother does not necessarily produce an anorexic daughter. That it is far more complicated than that. We discussed blame, guilt and shame and we really need to put those emotions aside and concentrate on helping their daughter. We reassured them that we were not blaming anyone and although motherly guilt is completely natural, that neither father nor mother should blame or feel guilty for their daughter's illness. We also talked in depth about particular personalities. Intelligent, perfectionists, sensitive and caring personalities that seemed more likely to suffer from eating disorders. Father then talked about his wife and that they were all the things he loved about her. Both parents said that what we had talked about described their daughter perfectly. The session was ended very differently to how it had started. Allowing both parent to talk openly enabled them to discuss their emotions, us to share what we knew, and them to think together about eating disorders, it helped them to reach a shared understanding and went some way to lessen the burden of blame and guilt. In many ways we were following guidelines, exploring the family's understanding of eating problems and providing psycho-education to help them better understand what their daughter (and in this case the mother) were going through, but the use of therapeutic relationship building had allowed us to follow this line of action actually much quicker than if we had followed a purely medical model by searching for a precipitating factor for the onset of Annie's problems and then recommending that her mother seek her own help in the hope that Annie's problems would resolve as a result of this.

The following session was a second family session. Annie had brought her food diary and said she had struggled a lot with it but she had tried her best. Parents were clearly acting together more as a couple and appeared much happier. They told us that the previous session had been extremely helpful for both of them. We discussed Annie's struggles and applauded her efforts. We then began to talk about others with struggles with their eating and then explained what we referred to as 'the voice of anorexia'. We discussed its punishing voice, how some have had to bargain with it and how it is illogical but compelling. We wondered whether she could relate to any of this. Annie then said that yes, she had the same voice. She said it made no sense but she had to follow its directions. We explained how the voice seems overwhelmingly powerful on its own, but when we employ the voices of our parents, it loses its power over us. We asked her if she could draw this 'voice of anorexia' so we could see how menacing it looked and asked her if she could enrol the help of her parents when the voice was telling her what she could and could not eat. We shared the words of the young woman with the traffic light analogy from Peggy Claude-Pierre's book (ibid) and how her mother helped her to battle that voice with her own louder, more logical voice. We reflected that this was a voice of someone who loved her daughter at a time when her daughter was struggling to love herself. Both parents said they would be Annie's external voice. We ended the session with another request for a food diary and a record of her ongoing struggles.

Annie returned the following week with an amazing drawing of the 'voice of anorexia'. It was a cross between a devil and a monster, and was a very scary image. Rather than concentrating on the food diary, we spent time looking at the drawing together and exploring it's meaning. Annie had clearly spent a great deal of time on this drawing and to her this was the demon that was fuelling the anorexia. We remarked on how frightening the drawing was, how wonderfully Annie had captured the essence of the demon and between us, therapists and parents, we all agreed that this was the stuff of nightmares which would have the same effect on us if it was attacking us. We were in fact normalising Annie's behaviour and externalizing the compulsion. We were joining with her and acknowledging her fears. We were not dismissing her battles with anorexia, we were not suggesting that it was all irrational. This empathic and non-blaming approach was so important. What we had to do was to comfort her, join with her and above all, reassure her that she would no longer be expected to battle this monster alone. We photocopied the picture and put the copy on the wall during the session. We asked Annie where she would like the drawing to be put in the house. She suggested it would be best placed on the fridge in the kitchen. That way she would safest knowing that her parents would be constantly reminded what it was she was battling. It was then that we asked if we could see the food diary. She said it had been a little easier than before to fight the 'voice of anorexia'. We asked what she felt had made it slightly easier. She told us it was knowing that she was not the only one with this voice, that others understood what she going through and drawing the demon helped her to visualise what she was fighting. Knowing she did not have to obey this demon had also helped. Prior to weighing her again, we asked what foods she had missed eating most. She said ice cream and Sunday roasts. After discussing her favourite flavours and the roast she missed the most, we ended the session suggesting if she thought about other foods she had missed, to tell her parents and perhaps they could go shopping together so she could choose herself.

Annie progressed quite quickly after this and returned to a more normal pattern of eating. Her age and developmental stage was a significant factor in her recovery, and she had quickly understood the externalization which enabled her to start to think differently about her eating. Trust and respect were vital in her recovery, but the way in which we had been able to work with the family to overcome the terrible silence that fell when we first talked about eating problems and addressed the 'elephant in the room' had been vital. By taking a non-judgemental and empathic stand we had developed a therapeutic relationship which then enabled parents to understand and support each other and Annie.

Case Study Two: Betty

A very different young person we saw was a 15 year old girl. We saw her together with her 17 year old sister and both her parents. The family were proudly of working class background, father was a factory worker, and mother was a 'stay at home mum'. We heard that maternal grandmother had passed away almost a year beforehand. The family were very close, and the Grandmother was, in mother's words, 'the glue that held the family together'. There were lots of tears when the family spoke of grandmother, she had apparently been a jolly woman who was kind, caring and astute, and had answers for everyone's problems, so the family seemed lost without her. She had been diagnosed with cancer and less than a year after her diagnosis has passed away.

Betty lost her appetite following her grandmothers death and had never got it back. When we weighed her we calculated that her BMI was 14 so she was both very thin and very sad. We talked about the 'voice of anorexia' and Betty was able to relate to this, and said she did have a voice instructing her to starve herself. She said she felt ok about this because she did not deserve to live and she wanted to join her grandmother. Upon hearing this, everyone in the family began to cry again. The grief in the room was palpable. We explained the assessment process and asked permission to delve into her background, explaining to her too that she may discover some lovely aspects of her early development. So that the older daughter would not feel left out, we asked about both young women. We were then taken on a trip down the family's memory lane. Parents talked about how they met, to the delight of the girls. Both parents giggled as they shared memories and the girls giggled too. The whole room lit up as they spoke. We saw what used to be a funny happy family before the death of grandmother and this joviality remained as parents talked about early development of both girls. The girls chipped in as we heard funny childhood stories whilst they all laughed together.

From this we discovered that there were no concerns regarding early milestones, no eating issues, no separation difficulties and a closeness of all family members. When we asked about food intake, Betty just said she had no appetite and agreed with the voice that was telling her to eat less and less. Everyone else agreed that she used to eat like a horse and that she had 'hollow legs'. Mum said that the only thing she would eat without being nagged these days was a McDonald's chicken nugget 'Happy Meal'. Parents explained that they were on a very tight budget and could not afford to pay for that every day so it was just a weekly treat. Betty refused to eat shop bought or home cooked nuggets unfortunately! We then asked if we could play a little game, one that we often did when a family have lost an important member. The family agreed and we brought another chair into the room. This was to be grandmother's chair. We told the family that when we are struggling with a loss of this enormity, we can forget what that person has taught us yet we all retain that persons voice in our heads.

We began with Betty. We asked her "what would grandmother say about you thinking that the best option is to starve yourself to death to be with her?" After giving this some thought, Betty laughed and said grandmother would tell her 'not to sound so bloody silly!'. We asked her to elaborate. She said grandmother would say she was being selfish and was not thinking about her parents and sister. There were more tears from everyone in the room as Betty decided that grandmother would want her to grow up and make something of her life. After going round the room and providing everyone the space to tell us what grandmother might say to them, we were able to return to Betty and ask her what she would like her mum to cook for her. She made a couple of suggestions after acknowledging that her parents could not afford to buy her McDonald's more than once a week and we agreed to meet the following week. After the session we spoke to the consultant who agreed to prescribe Betty antidepressants on the basis of our assessment of her mood. We decided to do home visits after that because of the time and expense to the family of coming to us, and made sure the appointments were after school and worked around fathers shifts. Progress was slow at first because even with (the memory of) grandmother on her side, the 'voice of anorexia' became more punishing and cruel. We would spent roughly half of each session on grief work for everyone, and the other half on Betty's food and voice diary. Slowly but surely, Betty began to become stronger in her fight against the voice. We encouraged her to take part in any activities that would give her pleasure. Betty began to go out with her friends more and found a boyfriend who delighted in taking her to McDonald's from time to time. She began to put on more weight and the voice got quieter and quieter until she was able to ignore it completely.

This family was very different to Annie's family, the precipitating factor here was clearly grief. Although this was a working class family with little money they had a closeness that enable them to work on their shared grief and change the family dynamic. It seemed that, as Betty lost weight her thoughts became more entrenched, and then the voice of anorexia took over and became the driver for more weight loss. We used a variation of externalisation again, the 'empty chair' to represent Grandmother, and restore the memory of her wisdom to help start to reverse that thinking process. However it was again important that we were able to engage the family sufficiently to help them in thinking differently.

Case Study Three: Connie

A third young person we saw was a 13 year old girl. Her father was in the armed forces and the family had travelled a lot as a result of his deployments. Living with her parents in several different countries over the years, Connie was an only child who was sensitive and quiet. Her eating difficulties had begun a year or so prior to being referred to our service. She had begun to restrict her intake by omitting certain foods from her diet. She became initially pescatarian, then vegetarian, and then vegan. Initially, her mother believed that these choices were due to animal welfare concerns but sought help after noticing what had turned into rapid weight loss in her daughter. Father was away on deployment abroad during the time we saw them so we only saw mother and daughter.

The initial assessment process turned up nothing remarkable. There was no apparent bullying and Connie was doing well at school and enjoying herself. Connie could not explain why she was eating so little. At the time, we first met her she was just eating one roast tomato and one roast onion a day. She loved to cook and bake with and for her mother but would not eat any of her creations. We decided to share what we had discovered when working with other young people with Connie and her mother. Upon finding out that she was not alone in her fight and that we could relate to her battles, Connie began to open up about her difficulties. Due to her low weight (she had a BMI of 14.5), the 'voice of anorexia' was very powerful. We encouraged Connie to allow us to weigh her backwards (we asked her to step onto the scales backwards so she could not see how much she weighed each time) to prevent the voice from becoming stronger. Connie seemed ashamed of this punishing voice and was believing everything it was telling her, that her parents did not love her, that she was ugly and worthless, and would never amount to anything.

We had to take it very slowly with Connie because she was really struggling with her thoughts. We would use sessions to talk about what she had cooked the week beforehand and talked about how we felt her hunger. We also got Connie and her mother to tell us about their travels, the good and not so good memories. We brought a lot of humour into the sessions and encouraged them both to tell us funny stories from their adventures. We also discussed her limited diet. Her mother had bought her a pet rabbit and although we all agreed that a roasted tomato and onion sounded delicious, Connie had to accept logically that she was eating less than the pet rabbit and that she was actually much bigger than the rabbit, so should probably be eating more than it was. Slowly, we managed to get Connie to eat more and more variety, and eventually she agreed to talk to a dietitian.

We asked Connie if she would bake for us too, and she was happy to do so. She brought in the most delicious cookies and cakes. We ate them in the room, remarking on how good they tasted. This allowed us to ask very gently what it was stopping her from having just a tiny bite. Going with the opening, we again used humour. We asked how would she know that her baking was tasty? She said it was because everyone said it was. We brought in the 'voice of anorexia' and reminded her it was telling her lies so maybe we were too? The mood was light and we asked if she was not the least bit curious? She laughed and took the tiniest bite of a cookie. She moved it around her mouth so slowly as if she was savouring each taste sensation. She then had to agree that we were telling the truth and she was in fact an exceptional cook. This was a real turning point, and the following week, Connie came in with her mother with a huge smile on her face. She had been shopping with her mother and they stopped for coffee. Connie had water but she had shared a chocolate chip muffin with her mother. Her recovery remained slow but what we did was to subtly re-engage her brain to discover how enjoyable food was. We had promised her we would never make her fat and that we together with her mother would just work towards getting her healthy again. Bit by bit, Connie began to talk about the foods that she used to enjoy and slowly she agreed to accept more and more in her diet. The voice of anorexia had become so strong and overpowering that she had to be allowed the time to trust other voices again. We were spending lots of time asking her about what she wanted, what she liked and what she needed. She had lost the ability to think for herself and believe she was worthy so we were really encouraging her back to herself.

Even though we were weighing her each session, we never discussed her weight with her, and with the backwards weighing that she allowed us to do, she did not know whether she was gaining weight. Connie had agreed that knowing this (her actual weight) would only give the voice of anorexia more ammunition against her. Instead, she entrusted that burden to us. She continued to bake for us and we would all eat together. We discussed the ingredients, and methods of baking, but specifically not the eating of the food. Connie began to go out with her friends on base more and she began to engage in more teenage appropriate activities, like sleeping over at friend's houses, having friends to stay over at her house, going to the cinema and eating takeaway pizza. Our sessions went from weekly to fortnightly and slowly became further and further apart. We kept our promise of support until it was no longer needed. Whilst we used some similar techniques with Connie the issue of trust was central to this relationship, and the relationship allowed us to use a lot of good-natured humour to help her move on.

Case Study Four: Delia

The following referral taught us that neurodevelopmentally challenged young people need not be harder to treat, despite many clinicians worrying that having comorbid conditions makes the task much more difficult (Kinnaird et al. 2017). Fourteen year old Delia had an autistic spectrum disorder (ASD) diagnosis. Having been teased at school about being plump, she had set out to diet and found out that like most things, when she put her mind to it, she got quite good at it. A high achiever, a perfectionist and with traits of OCD that could also be understood in the context of ASD, Delia was very concrete in her thinking. She researched how to lose weight and followed a diet plan religiously. Having lost what her parents described as her puppy fat, Delia was so pleased with her new slim form that she decided to see just how slim she could get. Mother blamed the fashion magazines that Delia was now obsessed with and the clearly underweight models. She was no longer being bullied but was admired by her peers for the weight she had lost, so Delia began to buy smaller and smaller sized clothes. Her protective parents, glad that she was fitting in better at school and seeming much happier at home, allowed her to continue on her quest until one day, mother saw Delia getting dressed and suddenly realised just how painfully thin she had got. No amount of talking to or cajoling would encourage Delia to stop her diet. By the time the parents took her to see the GP, Delia had shrunk to a (UK dress) size 6 and had a BMI of 14.

When we saw Delia, she was adamant that she had no desire to change her eating habits. She had gained so much by losing weight. She had friends and admirers and could fit into all the clothes she had always wanted to. When asked about the voice of anorexia, she admitted to having the voice but insisted that it was her helpful voice. It had helped her to diet and kept her on track when she had wanted to falter and encouraged her to continue to lose weight. Her parents were at a loss. There was a history of ASD in both father and mother's side of the family but in their relatives they were only with associated learning difficulties, so neither were able to make sense of their daughter's very different 'high-functioning' autism. As practitioners, we were also initially at a loss. Every inroad we tried to make Delia was able to block with her own logic. We then had to think about the ASD. We had to find a way into her mind and match her logic with life-preserving logical thinking. So we asked Delia to take her food diary and do some research of her own, so she could find out some things for herself, as we thought she was more likely to accept the facts that she was able to discover for herself, than listen to what we told her. Her task for that week was to compare her own food diary with what her research suggested was a complete diet for a healthy adult and also for a growing young person like her. We also suggested she find out what was a healthy weight for her height. Delia delighted at this task.

She returned the following week a very different young person to the one we had been seeing. She now knew that although the diet had been helpful in losing weight, she had taken it too far and was now very underweight and this was affecting her growth, her development and her brain function. She spent the entire session talking about her newfound knowledge and all the changes she had already made to become healthy again. Rather than us giving her and the family a session of psychoeducation on nutrition and the effects of limited food intake we encouraged her to find this out for herself, which was much more acceptable for her. Unlike the other young people who had experienced a very punishing voice, she had understood hers as being helpful and supportive. When she started to alter her eating patterns, the voice told her not to, but her very logical brain was able to tell the voice she was not dieting any more and she was able to combat it on that very concrete level.

Once Delia had turned the corner through her own research, and had discovered the facts for herself, rather than dismissing everything we had been saying, her recovery was swift. Her parents were relieved (as were we!) and Delia continued with her life, though she had very little insight into just how poorly she had been.

Case Study Five: Elaine

The next case was difficult for very different reasons. Elaine was a 16 year old girl. She was the daughter of two well-educated professionals. She had a younger sister, and both girls were very intelligent, and attended private schools. Elaine was sensitive and introverted in nature whilst her sister was outgoing and sociable. There was nothing remarkable in Elaine's developmental history but she had a BMI of 15 when we met her. The family were affluent, and the girls had enjoyed holidays abroad and around Britain with their parents. Each family member played musical instruments and there was a wide network of family friends so they all maintained a busy work and social life. Both parents had moved to pursue their careers, so the extended families were living in other parts of the UK. Both parents had successful full-time careers and were equally respected in their fields.

At the time of referral, we were without a medical consultant in our outpatient team. This was problematic for the parents because not having a medical consultant to oversee their daughter's treatment was interpreted by them as receiving an inferior service. This in itself hindered the relationship we were trying to build with the family. Despite specialist dietetic input, family and individual sessions, Elaine continued to lose weight. After a few months of slow but steady weight loss, Elaine's BMI had dropped to 13.5. We therefore had to begin discussions with the family about admission to an inpatient unit. A specialist unit was found in another county and Elaine was admitted for assessment. She initially made good progress and her BMI rose back to 15. Elaine then negotiated with the staff that she should begin to manage her own intake. Unfortunately, Elaine's BMI did not get higher than 15.5

over the following few months within the unit, but it was negotiated that Elaine should return home and access services from our local outreach team.

Therapy remained a struggle, with Elaine reluctant to engage and parents rapidly losing the little faith they had in the service. Knowing that any drop in her BMI could result in a further admission, Elaine managed to maintain a BMI of 15.5 for the duration and was eventually transferred on to adult services. This relationship had never really got to the point where Elaine and her family were fully able to trust us because what we were able to provide was not what they wanted and needed. For all the importance we put on therapeutic relationships the expectation of an expert medical model (which they did receive later in the course of treatment) had not been met in those crucial early stages of engagement.

Case Study Six: Felicity
The following case was even trickier. We met a young woman aged 16 years with her parents for an initial assessment. She had a younger sibling who had chosen to stay at home. Following the introductions, before we could begin to talk about the assessment process, the parents told us their daughter was not eating and was now averse even to drinking. We asked Felicity how much she had drunk that day. She said nothing and parents confirmed that she had not drunk anything at all for the previous 3 days either. When asked why, she said that even drinking water was going to make her put on weight. We explained to Felicity and her family that not drinking anything was in fact life threatening and then said we would have to halt the session and ask for advice. We phoned our own inpatient unit and spoke to the consultant. We explained we were yet to begin our assessment but had been told something very concerning. The consultant asked us to bring the family over to the unit (which was on the same site). After hearing from the family and this being confirmed by Felicity, the consultant did a quick skin test and confirmed that she was indeed dehydrated. He suggested an emergency admission to the unit. This came as a complete shock to Felicity and her family. Even though they wanted time to digest what was happening and initially refused the admission, the consultant explained that this was actually a life-threatening situation and that if they refused, Felicity would have to be sectioned under the Mental Health Act and admitted compulsorily to the unit. The parents and Felicity reluctantly agreed to an informal admission, which took place immediately.

What happened following this was in fact quite tragic. Felicity once admitted, refused to allow anything to pass her lips. She had to be restrained and tube fed. We tried to meet with Felicity and her family to complete our assessment on several occasions during her admission but were unable to get anywhere. Felicity was restrained and fed with a nasogastric tube three times a day for the following month. She had shut down completely and she remained adamant that nothing would willingly pass her lips. Her parents had shut down too. Any relationship we tried to develop with Felicity and her parents was thwarted. Despite our best attempts to remain nonjudgmental we eventually began to assume that the parents were hiding some dark secret as we tried and tried, to no avail, to connect with them on any level. Felicity was transferred to a unit many miles away that worked specifically with anorexia[2] in the hopes that she would begin to eat willingly again and parents remained distant with us. When Felicity returned to the local unit 6 months later, we tried to resume therapy sessions with the family again, but they only engaged on a superficial level.

Felicity only remained at the local unit for a short time before she was discharged. We continued with our efforts to talk about fun and enjoyable times she had had with her family in the past and tried to make roads into a working relationship with the family. Up until this point, Felicity was passively following the food plan given to her by the dietitian. She was now a technically healthier BMI of 16 but we did not feel we had any real connection to her or her thoughts, or the thoughts or feelings of her parents, and we had only met her sibling once in the whole time we were involved with the family.

One incident particularly sticks out. During one session when we were trying to help her to connect with her past enjoyment of food, she told us that she was going out for a meal with her family later on that day. We asked her what food choices she would like to make. She began to ask if she could have pizza. We said of course she could. She then asked if she could have a burger. We said of course she could. She then asked if she could have a really juicy burger. We said of course. Having reiterated over and over again in the past that we and her parents would never let her over eat, we set the date for the following session. This was cancelled by the family as was the next session. During the following week, prior to the agreed session, we had a phone call from the mother. Felicity has eaten the burger the night they went out, plus fries and a huge dessert. Since then, she had not stopped eating. She was locking herself in her bedroom with huge amounts of food and eating everything she could get hold of. We did a home visit and found Felicity locked in her bedroom refusing to come down. We reminded her parents that together we had promised Felicity that we would not let her do this. We tried to find a way forward with the family to help Felicity to eat her way back to health gradually and talked about the chance that without careful boundaries, this could turn into a different sort of eating problem, bulimia. Her parents were cross with us, however, and just wanted their daughter to eat what she wanted. Unfortunately, without the conversations and support needed to regulate her food intake, Felicity continued to binge. As her weight began to balloon, purging began and soon, Felicity had indeed acquired a different eating disorder. In this case, without a trusting relationship to enable us to understand how she was thinking and help her to make planned changes, we had become

---

[2] At the time of this case our local services had a general CAMHS in-patient unit on the same campus as the community service. Since this time the unit has expanded and also has a purpose-built specialist Eating Disorders facility, but back then we still had to send young people a long way from home for specialist treatment.

part of a system which treated symptoms without being able to look at the underlying causes for those symptoms.

8.4 Bulimia Nervosa

Bulimia Nervosa tends to be diagnosed in those who binge and then purge. It typically involves consuming large amounts of food very quickly and then using various methods to purge the body of the calories (RCPsych 2019). This can take the form of vomiting, abuse of laxatives, intensive exercise or periods of starvation. Often sufferers describe an intense hunger which causes them to eat rapidly until they can eat no more followed by self-hate and disgust which leads them to attempt to purge the body as quickly as possible. Some may binge for weeks followed by weeks of self-starvation. Others may binge and induce vomiting straight after. The risks to health are just as dangerous as those with anorexia and although it can be better hidden, sufferers can be just as secretive as they battle the internal negative voices that keep them chained to the disorder.

Case Study Seven: Gina
A 17 year old young woman was referred to us by her GP. She had attended the surgery without her parents' knowledge and explained she had been bingeing and purging for the past 2 years and she wanted help. It is quite unusual for a young person to be referred without the knowledge of their parents but as this was a family well known to the GP and she was only 6 months below the age of 18, the GP was happy to refer her. In team the allocation meeting, it was decided that the young woman was Gillick competent (Larcher and Hutchinson 2008) and as long as it was made clear that we would be legally and ethically obliged to inform her parents and others should we become concerned that she cause harm to herself or to others, then we would comply with her wishes. This case was therefore unusual for us on two fronts. Usually, parents become concerned about the mental health of their child or young person and take them to see the GP who then refers on to us. The young person being referred is not (legally and developmentally) an autonomous being and often does not believe they are experiencing any difficulties at all. This was not only, in essence, a self-referral but the young person was not only aware of her difficulties, but actively wanting help with them.

Gina could be described as a little overweight, with a BMI of just under 28. She had clearly spent a lot of time on her appearance and make up. She smiled when we met her and greeted us in a very mature manner. Under these circumstances, we decided not to begin with a full developmental assessment. Instead, we asked Gina to tell us her story and what had brought her to therapy at this time. Gina described herself as a failed dieter. She had been trying to control her eating for almost 3 years but could only manage to restrict her food intake a month at a time. Following this she would experience huge cravings and begin to consume large quantities of all the foods she had craved. She would then experience shame and began a pattern of vomiting when she felt she had eaten too much. She had done this in secret and as far as she was aware, no one else knew what she was doing. Gina had known that what she was doing was not the right way to go about it but had kept telling herself that when the time was right, she would change. But the time never seemed right and instead she had got stuck in this pattern of binging and purging. Gina had been offered a place at university, subject to her obtaining the predicted grades, but what had caused her to seek help now was a television programme on bulimia. Through the documentary she watched, Gina discovered that vomiting over a prolonged period of time not only completely rots teeth, but also has major physical health implications. It was then that she realised she needed help to overcome this disorder and she wanted to do this before she went to live independently at university.

We decided that the first thing we should do was to offer more psychoeducation on bulimia, as this was what had prompted her to seek help. We explained that from the first bite, the body begins to digest the food in the stomach therefore vomiting after binging brings back mainly stomach acids and little food. Likewise, purging by way of laxatives does the same thing. Instead of ridding the body of the food, it just disrupts the workings of the intestinal tract. We also talked about the voice that can become the driver for eating disorders. Gina told us about her own voice that only allowed her to binge if she vomited after and how it also constantly told her that she was fat and unlovable and that she was a failure at dieting. We spent time discussing Gina's own voice and what it was telling her. We asked permission to help with a two-pronged attack. We suggested we look at her body image, what precipitating the bulimia, alongside what the voice was saying and how to help her to regulate her eating at the same time. Gina agreed to this approach, so we asked her to go home and eat as normally as possible. We clarified with her that this meant no dieting and no bingeing, and to return the following week with a food diary including her thought patterns and specifically what the voice was saying during and after each meal. The psychoeducation we provided gave Gina trust in what we were saying, and she left the session appearing much happier than when the session began.

When Gina returned, she had done everything we asked of her. She had found it much easier to not binge than she had thought she would. Her diary had been carefully completed and detailed what she ate and how she felt about it. She also described her inner thoughts and instead of listening to them and believing them, she was telling herself she was now on the road to recovery and she would not let them dictate to her any more. We discussed how the bulimia began with her trying to diet but just could not just keep it up and then got into this unhealthy pattern because she thought it was working for her. Now she had more information, she felt she had more control over the bulimia. Over the next few sessions, Gina was able to eat without bingeing, which in turn took away the need to purge, and she was visibly happier. Gina came to us determined to address and beat her eating disorder. She had needed a nurturing, compassionate non-judgmental approach and a little more information on the drivers and maintainers of her eating disorder. With this, she was able to take herself forward, with relatively little help, but help that had been centred on her needs and provided in a way which she was able to accept and use.

Case Study Eight: Helen

Helen, aged 13, was referred to us because her mother had discovered countless bags of what looked like food that had been chewed and spat out in Helen's wardrobe. She then looked further and found more bags concealed under the bed and in the drawers. She took Helen to the GP and the family subsequently brought her to us. Helen was of average BMI but small in stature, as were her parents and sister who was a year older. We asked who would like to start telling us what had brought them to us and Helen's mother began to tell us their story. Helen looked embarrassed by what her mother was saying. Upon noticing this, we began a conversation between ourselves. We remarked upon the amount of self-control needed to do something like this and both agreed we did not have anywhere near that level of self-control. We spoke to Helen and explained we had not come across this before so we would love for her to tell us in detail so we could better help others who may do this too. This not only made Helen feel at ease but by putting her in the expert position and expressing genuine curiosity, Helen opened up to us. Technically this was a variation on a systemic psychotherapy tool known as the reflecting team (Anderson 1987), in this case the co-therapists taking a moment to talk to each other about their reactions to what the family were telling us, rather than having a separate team to do this. It is effective only when used in a spirit of genuine curiosity to free up a conversational standpoint which has the potential to become stuck or end up leading down a therapeutic blind alley. So we expressed amazement at how she managed to do this and after she explained how, we used humour to encourage her to talk freely and discovered that she even managed to do it with chocolate. We decided together to call it 'chew and spit', rather than jumping into categorizing it as bulimic behaviour or as an illness. We asked what led up to this behaviour and how she came up with such a novel idea? She said she had wanted to eat whatever she wanted without putting on weight and that is how she came up with the idea. We discussed her fear of putting on weight and where it had come from. Other girls at school had become obsessed with their weight and were dieting. Helen became fearful that unless she took measures to prevent it happening to her then she may become fat and be rejected by her peers.

We said we could understand how she got to thinking like that, however she shared the same build as her parents and sister. We then gave both parents and Helen's sister individual time within the session to tell us about what methods they used to stay the weight they were. No one else in the family had ever dieted. In fact, Helen's mother and father each had slim parents and naturally slim siblings. Because we had used humour to develop a trusting relationship within the session and this was a family that liked humour, and joined us in this spirit, there was quite a good amount of joviality when everyone was sharing this history with us. We felt comfortable, and judged it was appropriate to continue with this approach (despite the seriousness of the situation) when asking Helen where she had got the idea that she might get fat. Helen said she had assumed that other family members might have their own secret ways of staying slim. We asked if she knew that in just spitting out what she had already chewed, she was not really altering her calorie intake, and she had not realised that. We asked her permission to test it out with an experiment that she could do between sessions. We suggested we weigh her at this first session and she go home and not spit anything out for a week and when she returned, we would weigh her again and measure the difference. Then she could spend the following week chewing and spitting and when she returned, we would weigh her again and discuss what we discovered together. Helen liked the idea of this experiment, and happily complied. After the first week, there was no change to her weight, and she seemed a little surprised at this. The following week (during which she returned to the 'chew and spit' habit) there was still no change in her weight. Again, Helen was surprised by the outcome of our co-constructed experiment. We did spend time over these sessions getting to know more about the family, find out their interests and their hobbies, and developing a trusting relationship. We encouraged them to do more of what they enjoyed doing together and, again rather playfully, we also got to find out what were the hardest foods to chew and spit and what were the easiest. Helen told us that chocolate and ice-cream were the hardest. As a consequence of the results of our experiment, Helen asked, "Does that mean I can eat ice-cream and chocolates again without spitting out what's left?"

It would have been relatively easy to have been shocked by the strange behaviour that brought Helen and her family to us, and to react to their shock and shame in the initial conversation and taken this case down a much different route. Fortunately, we were able to use our curiosity about how this unusual pattern of behaviour had developed, we picked up on the way in which the family dealt with difficult emotions, and build on this by using an appropriate level of humour to develop a trusting relationship. As with some of our previous interventions we used some psychoeducation and systemic psychotherapy techniques, but the progress was made because we were able to establish a rapport with the individual and the family which enabled them to conduct the behavioural experiment which led to a discovery that the technique Helen had developed actually was pointless, and that she did not need to continue to do this. The uncovering for her that her genetics meant she probably did not need to diet (as she discovered that the rest of the family remained naturally slim) was the other part of the puzzle, and she soon returned to a normal pattern of eating.

8.5   Orthorexia Nervosa

Orthorexia nervosa has only been understood better in recent years (Dunn and Bratman 2016). Whilst it is not commonly seen in under 18s, it can still be found in teenagers. Orthorexia can be harder to diagnose because it is an extension of an interest in healthy eating which becomes an obsessive compulsion to restrict the diet to what are deemed as healthy foods. It differs from some of the other eating problems which usually focus on quantity of food, instead focusing on quality of food, but often with similar outcomes. An orthorexia sufferer will likely omit all fats, cheese and often dairy from their diet whilst calorie counting and vigorously exercising. Eating is no longer for pleasure but purely to sustain what they see as a healthy body. Young people will typically be underweight but not enough to be seen as critical, as is typical of anorexia, so this can easily be missed by healthcare professionals. The desire to keep to a healthy diet can be seen as logical, and something we more normally wish to promote. The negative thought pattern in orthorexia which also feeds the other eating disorders, however, is still alive and present in orthorexia and similarly needs addressing if it is proving detrimental to the health of the individual.

Case Study Nine: Ivan
A 16 year old young man was referred to us by his GP because of his distorted body image. His parents were aware of the referral, but complied to his wishes that he be seen alone. Ivan had a BMI of 16, he explained that he was observing a strict healthy diet, lots of vegetables, low fat foods, nuts and grains with some but not much meat. He had been trying to obtain a more muscular body and had been working out at the gym each day but was just getting thinner. He was disheartened by all of this effort and was very saddened by his failure. He discussed his low mood with us openly, focusing on his irritability, tearfulness, negative thinking and his difficulties with sleeping. Ivan said he had been experiencing these symptoms for at least 6 months. We spoke to the medical consultant who prescribed antidepressants, which he was happy to take. We discussed with him the difference between dieting and trying to get a 'weight lifter's body' and explained that he just was not eating enough to maintain the thin physique he had and manage the excessive exercise regime he was undertaking. We asked him to keep a food diary and a calculation of his calories so we could get to know more about his eating patterns. We also suggested that he refrain from exercise until we helped him to attain a healthier weight.

When he returned for the second session, he talked about the difficulties he had had in stopping exercise. A part of his brain was telling him he had to exercise otherwise he was failing. He had completed his food diary and had calculated his calories and knew, logically, that he was not eating enough. We told him that we had found that often with eating difficulties and disorders, those suffering tended to have a powerful overriding voice compelling them to continue on a particular course even when they have found evidence that the course that they are following is detrimental to their health. Ivan became quite tearful at this stage and talked about feeling lost and helpless. We asked about a time when he remembered being happier and who he had around him to help him to fight this internal voice. Ivan felt his mother could help, so he agreed to discuss the session with her, and let her know he would need her support. We wondered with him whether a thought diary might help (another CBT technique), and he agreed that writing down these thoughts may also help to diminish their power over him. Over the next few sessions we helped Ivan to battle these thoughts. Slowly he gained more control over them and was able to eat what he needed to gain the weight. He used information from the internet to gain more information about what he needed to do and to eat in order to obtain the body he desired and slowly the internal voices were beaten. Again we took the time to engage Ivan so that he trusted us enough to use our suggestions to challenge the thoughts. The medication also helped, but a tickbox approach of medication, and psychoeducation without taking time to develop a trusting therapeutic relationship would most likely have been rejected by the internal voice that was initially overriding the logical part of his brain.

Case Study Ten: Jack
Another young man we saw was aged 15, and had battled OCD in the past. He was actually pleased that the OCD voice had converted itself into what he saw as a logical voice that told him to eat healthily and exercise. This was something he enjoyed doing, and despite his low weight (he had a BMI of 17) as far as he was concerned, he was a little thin but had nothing to worry about. He prided himself on his strength and determination and was very happy that he had the power to refuse to eat anything unhealthy and to exercise regularly. He did not see his weight or lifestyle, as he called it, anything to worry about and felt that those around him, including his parents, were worrying about nothing. Despite lengthy intervention, he was not able to shift his thinking or even to acknowledge that it might be slightly flawed.

This young man simply was not ready to change. Jack was happy with his food choices and with his level of exercise. We had a very close trusting relationship with both him and his parents, having been involved in treating his OCD previously, and there was honesty and respect. He was a lovely sensitive, and usually compliant young man. He was just so wedded to his own ideas of what was and what was not healthy living that he was unable to accept he may need help. In this case the voice defied all our attempts to shift Jack's thinking to a more balanced view of healthy eating and lifestyle.

8.6 Summary

In conclusion, the nursing skills that we discussed at the beginning were crucial for the recovery of each of those we were able to help. These are skills that most would say they use regularly, but to be able to apply them consistently is a skill in itself. Being able to not fall into the trap of automatically searching for, and concentrating on potential causes is hard, because we naturally want to 'fix' things. Instead it is important to remember to look for ways to treat, and help recovery, based on what is discovered about the young person and the family. It goes beyond the belief that we are showing empathy, and into actually being able to put ourselves in the shoes of each family member and to spend time wondering how we would think and feel were this have happened to us and our family.

We need to be able to think about what would make us feel not just listened to but heard. Families we worked with told us that they felt their feelings were not only acknowledged but also understood and respected. It is vital that we go deeper and enable each family member to feel like they are treated and valued as individuals but also as part of the collective family group. We need to bear in mind that this journey the family has been on together may have evoked feelings of shame, guilt and inadequacy. We also need to remember that not being able to feed and nurture a child can be one of the most painful experiences a parent can go through.

Above all, as we embark upon this journey with the child or young person and their family, we should keep in mind that we are becoming part of their story. It can evolve into a story whereby each family member looks back at a time when professionals saw them through their darkest moments, who nurtured and cared for them or a time when they were in the most need, those put there to help them, had turned their experience into a nightmare.

Having said this, we cannot help everyone who comes through our doors, and we have deliberately included some case studies which were less successful in terms of outcomes. Some are just not ready to change, and some are not provided with what they perceive to be the right kind of care. Others experience what they feel to be a nightmare right at the beginning of their journey and lose trust in everyone else they come into contact with. But when, as professionals, we take everything into consideration, age, development, and family experiences, we can use the skills we have sensitively and with compassion so each family member feels listened to and valued. It sounds like a simple thing, but it can be difficult to actually enact in a pressurised healthcare system, so we have taken the time to try and illustrate what it actually takes to integrate this into nursing practice.

References

Anderson T (1987) The reflecting team: dialog and meta-dialog in clinical work. Fam Process 26:415–481

Boston P (2000) Systemic family therapy and the influence of post-modernism. Adv Psychiatr Treat 6:250–257

Claude-Pierre P (1997) The secret language of eating disorders. Random House Canada, Toronto

DAWBA (2012) Development and wellbeing assessment. https://www.dawba.info/a0.html. Accessed 1 March 2019

Dunn T, Bratman S (2016) On orthorexia nervosa: a review of the literature and proposed diagnostic criteria. Eat Behav 21:11–17

Eisler I et al (2016) Maudsley service manual for child and adolescent eating disorders. https://www.national.slam.nhs.uk/wp-content/uploads/2011/11/Maudsley-Service-Manual-for-Child-and-Adolescent-Eating-Disorders-July-2016.pdf. Accessed 1 March 2019

Halse C, Honey A, Broughtwood D (2007) The paradox of virtue: (re)thinking deviance, anorexia and schooling. Gend Educ 19(2):219–235

Kinnaird E, Norton C, Tchanturia K (2017) Clinician's views on working withanorexia nervosa and autistic spectrum disorder: a qualitative study. BMC Psychiatry 17:292

Kinsella P, Garland A (2008) Cognitive behavioural therapy for mental health workers: a beginner's guide. Routledge, Hove

Larcher V, Hutchinson A (2008) How should paediatricians assess Gillick competence? Arch Dis Child 95:305–307

McDougall et al (2017) Children and young people's mental health: essentials for nurses and other professionals. Routledge, Abingdon

NICE (2017) NICE guideline (NG69) eating disorders: recognition and treatment. NICE, London

RCPsych (2014) College report 189: MARSIPAN—management of really sick patients with anorexia nervosa. Royal College of Psychiatrists, London

RCPsych (2019) Information on anorexia and bulimia. https://www.rcpsych.ac.uk/mental-health/ problems-disorders/anorexia-and-bulimia. Accessed 1 March 2019

Rikani et al (2013) A critique of the literature on the etiology of eating disorders. Ann Neurosci 20(4):157–161

Smink FRE, van Hoeken D, Hoek HW (2012) Epidemiology of eating disorders: incidence, prevalence and mortality rates. Curr Psychiatry Rep 14(4):406–414

Wright LM, Leahey M (2013) Nurses and families: a guide to family assessment and intervention, 6th edn. FA Davis, Philadelphia

Chapter 9
Nurse or Psychotherapist? Using Nursing Skills in Therapeutic Relationships and Psychotherapies

Ann Marie Cox

9.1 Increased Use of Psychotherapies in CAMHS

The use of evidence-based therapies has rapidly increased in CAMHS over the last few years through the introduction of Children and Young People's Improving Access to Psychological Therapies (CYP-IAPT) (NHS England (NHSE) 2018a) in 2011. CYP-IAPT was initiated following the recommendations of the CAMHS review (2008) and the success of the adult IAPT programme (NHSE 2018b). CYP-IAPT embeds within its strategy, a rolling programme of clinical training in evidence-based therapies and interventions. This provides CAMHS clinicians with opportunity to train in an evidence-based therapy whilst continuing to work in clinical practice. The strategy aims to upskill the CAMHS workforce and increase access and availability of evidence-based therapies for children and young people (CYP), offering access to therapy at the right time and in the right place (NHSE 2018a). There are a number of training courses offered at different academic levels, which means that some professionals are trained in offering evidence-based interventions and others to therapist level. The CYP-IAPT strategy involves training partner agencies of CAMHS, such as social care, third sector agencies and education staff in evidence-based interventions; these services will usually sit at tier 2 or will be universal services. This aspect of the strategy endeavours to upskill the community workforce, that generally have involvement with CYP before they reach tier 3 specialist CAMHS, in an attempt to help CYP earlier and prevent the need for referral to specialist (tier 3) CAMHS (NHSE 2018a). In 2017, the Department of Health and Social Care (DHSC) and the Department of Education (DE) produced the green paper 'transforming children and young peoples mental health provision'. This detailed piloting the development of new mental health support teams as part of a national trailblazer involving 25 pilot sites in England (DHSC/DE 2018). These

A. M. Cox (✉)
North Staffordshire Combined NHS Trust, North Staffordshire, UK

© Springer Nature Switzerland AG 2020
L. Baldwin (ed.), *Nursing Skills for Children and Young People's Mental Health*,
https://doi.org/10.1007/978-3-030-18679-1_9

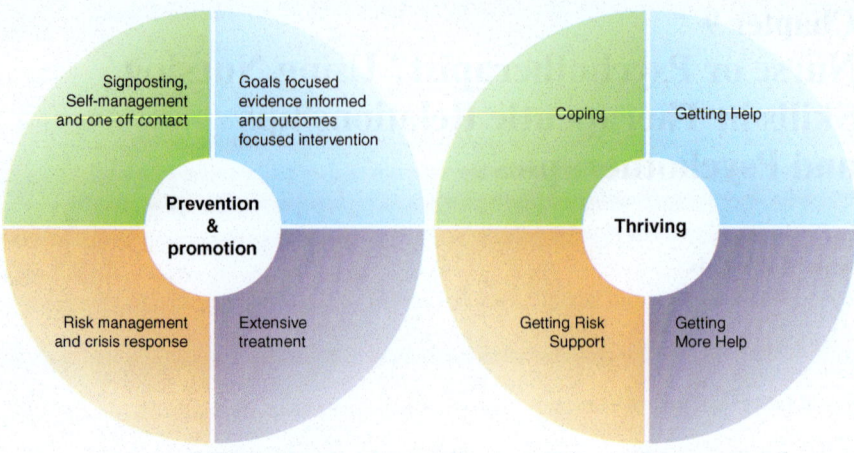

Fig. 9.1 The THRIVE model. (Wolpert et al. 2014:7)

teams are now in development and will concentrate on supporting education providers, their students and familes by offering evidence-based therapeutic interventions, with each team supporting up to 20 education establishments. This is alongside a 'core' offer of developing a well-being strategy and embedding positive mental health support in each establishment.

The staged level of therapeutic intervention offered by Tier 2 and Tier 3 services, relate to the Anna Freud Centre, THRIVE, Tavistock model of CAMHS (Wolpert et al. 2014). This relatively new model of CAMHS has been developed alongside CYP-IAPT in an attempt to better understand the needs of CYP from a service and business perspective. THRIVE aims to support CYP move through pathways more easily, having wrap-around care and aims to move away from the 'clunky' tiered approach to CAMHS. Tier 2 would generally map onto 'getting help' where more therapeutic interventions would be used and tier 3 onto 'getting more help' where psychotherapy would be used in working with more severe and enduring mental health problems. The Thrive model is embedded within the Future in Mind (Department of Health (DH) and NHS England 2015) strategy which continues to be one of the leading strategic documents for CAMHS in 2019. This chapter will discuss the scope of some evidence-based therapies and consider some of the interventions and skills that are used widely with CYP (Fig. 9.1).

Learning Point Summary
- CYP-IAPT has significantly increased access to psychological therapies over the last few years.
- CYP-IAPT aims to upskill clinicians in specialist CAMH services and those professionals that have significant contact with CYP in wider community services.
- The Department of Health and Social Care and the Department of Education are piloting mental health support teams using evidence-based therapeutic

interventions to support education providers in embedding their mental health and well-being strategies.

- There are different levels of training in evidence-based therapy.
- Evidence-based interventions can be offered by a nurse without any formal therapeutic training as long as it is informed by the evidence base and is supervised appropriately.

9.2   How Has Therapy Evolved?

It is important to have an understanding of the history of therapy and how it has developed over time, so that nurses can make an informed decision about why they may use a specific intervention or refer to the appropriate therapy. Each evidence-based therapy modality has an underpinning philosophy that defines its structure and process. We will consider some therapies and structures later in the chapter.

Understanding and treating human behavioural difficulties can be traced back to the ancient Greek philosophers such as Aristotle and Socrates (Robertson 2010). There was significant development of therapy in the nineteenth century, where mesmerism and hypnosis were dominant throughout the era (Robertson 2010). Walter Cooper Dendy an English psychiatrist developed the term *psychotherapeia* in his *book 'Psyche: A discourse on the birth and pilgrimage of thought' (1853)*. Dendy asserted that psychotherapeia could be used for numerous mental health difficulties including sorrow, distress, grief, anxiety and fear. Dendy considered the writings of the Greeks in great detail and argued that all emotional feelings had physiological impacts too, with examples such as depression simulating sedating medication effects and grief and fear reducing vascular action. Dendy argued that by using *psychotherpeia,* you could reduce or change the thoughts that are symptomatic in depression and fear, thus improving the patient's presentation (Dendy 1853).

Sigmund Freud further developed psychoanalysis at the turn of the twentieth century and developed his theories around trauma being related to childhood and sexual oppression in childhood (Rubovits-Seitz 2014). Freud believed, by working with the unconsciousness and where patients could freely associate, that he could reduce the emotional impact on the patient. Brown (1964:17–18) describes Freud as asking his patients to relax on the couch and close their eyes and verbalise about whatever should cross their minds, seemingly helping the patient connect with their unconsciousness and have free association. Freud, according to Brown (Ibid), believed that this verbalisation would allow for "painful emotions to be drained off as if it were a psychic abscess which had been opened and the purulent matter within it evacuated". Freud's work was significant as he conceptualised mental function operating separately from biological functions (Solms and Saling 1986). However, Freud was not alone in his development of psychic understanding, with theorists Pierre Janet, a psychical researcher (Evrard et al. 2018), Paul Dubois (1905) who wrote 'The psychic treatment of nervous disorders' and other researchers such as Hippolyte Bernheim, James Braid and Jean Martin Charcott were all purpo-sively developing the understanding about psychic phenomena (Wallace and Gach 2008). Criticisms were made about several of the psychoanalytical theories espe-cially from neurologists, who were concerned about the omission of any anatomical or physiological connections being made with the psychic disorders (Ibid). Freud's work has continued to be developed through psychodynamic therapy through semi-nal theorists such as Carl Jung (1959) and Melanie Klein (1960).

Further into the twentieth century, many behaviourist researchers were develop-ing their theories, with the most infamous of the time being Ivan Pavlov's classical conditioning theory, where he commanded dogs to salivate on being presented with a stimuli and Burrhus Skinner's operant conditioning theory, which demonstrated repeated, learned behaviours for the access of a reward (Mills 1998). Following the behaviourist's developments, came a wide range of evolving treatments for psychic phenomena. These ranged from Rational Emotive Behavioural Therapy (REBT) by Albert Ellis (1962) which is said to be the major precursor to the Cognitive and Behavioural Therapies (CBT) (Robertson 2010). REBT theory was further devel-oped by A.T. Beck's (1967) cognitive approach and J. Wolpe's (1969) behavioural approach. These developments were collaborated and demonstrate our more recent understanding of CBT. Concurrently, marriage therapies developed by Haley (1962) and Greene and Solomon (1963) blended into marriage and family therapy in the 1970s (Kaslow 2000), and further into family therapy throughout the 1980s influ-enced by seminal researchers such as John Howells (1971), Robin Skynner (1976) and John Byng-Hall (1982).

More recently, toward the twenty-first century, the third wave therapies such as acceptance and commitment therapy, mindfulness-based cognitive therapy, dialec-tical behavioural therapy, meta cognitive therapy and compassion focused therapy have been developed in a bid to move away from examining content and concen-trate on the relationship between concepts (Hayes and Hofmann 2017). Therapies continually develop with increased understanding about the pathology of disor-ders, human anatomy and physiology and the relationships between the mind and body. The development of therapies is also impacted on by environmental and systemic influencing factors including wider social and cultural change. There are a diverse range of therapies, each with an individual philosophical underpinning. It is important to have some understanding of these, so the right therapy can be offered to the right child, young person or family at the right time. Trained evi-dence-based therapists can help you understand what therapy will be useful for the given presentation. The National Institute of Health and Care Excellence (NICE) (2019) also offers guidance about what therapies are demonstrated to be effective for specific diagnoses. It is important to make an informed choice about what ther-apy you offer, as not all therapies are suitable for all people. This is due to the therapeutic framework of each therapy differing significantly. The next section offers detail about available therapies within CAMHS; this is followed by a discus-sion of some of the fundamental interventions that are central to all therapies and how best to perform these.

Learning Point Summary
- Psychotherapy or helping people deal with psychological difficulties can be traced back to the ancient Greeks.
- There are many different models of therapy.
- Therapy is always developing.
- It is really important to ensure the therapy is the right fit for the CYP and not the CYP be fitted for the therapy.
- NICE (2019) offers guidance about what therapies are demonstrated to be effective for specific diagnoses.
- Trained therapists can help you choose an appropriate therapy or intervention for a patient.

9.3 An Overview of Some of the Therapies

9.3.1 Cognitive Behavioural Therapy

Cognitive Behavioural Therapy (CBT), as previously discussed, was developed from the works of Albert Ellis (1962), A.T. Beck (1967) and J. Wolpe (1969). CBT is an evidence-based treatment for a number of mental health difficulties as indicated by NICE (2019). CBT is fundamentally based on the idea that thoughts have an impact on behaviours and vice versa. When explaining what CBT is to CYP, it is helpful to understand the words 'cognitive' and 'behavioural'; these are long words that CYP's dont always understand. In practice, it is helpful to ask if they know what CBT means, if they don't know, then explain each word clearly. Then help them understand how the model of CBT demonstrates the relationship between behaviours and thoughts. An example of this may be asking them what they would do and think if they saw a big spider; you can then relate their thoughts and behaviours in this situation, explaining how this is aligned to the CBT model; 'the spider is going to get me', therefore I 'scream' and 'run away'. As the CYP had the thought that the spider was going to get them, this then encouraged them to scream and get to safety by running away. You can explain to the CYP, if you were able to change the thought about the spider, not be scared of spiders or not thinking that the spider wants to get them, and then the behaviour of running away would subsequently change.

CBT also includes three more fundamental influences to the development of a problem, these being the physiology, or what is happening physically to the body, emotions and the environment the problem is related to (Westbrook et al. 2011). In our example of seeing the spider, the physiology may be increased heart rate and breathing, sweating, feeling tense; emotions may be scared, anxious, worried; the environment would change the response of the patient, for example if the patient is in the bathroom with the spider, this is very likely to be a different response if the patient saw spider in the garden or on the television, or if it was a toy or a picture of a spider (Steimer 2002). Within the CBT philosophy, there is an importance to understand the staged levels of thought processes, which include negative automatic thoughts, cognitive distortions, dysfunctional assumptions and core beliefs (Bennett-Levy et al. 2004).

CBT is a structured, time limited and brief therapy that holds collaboration with the patient central to its philosophy. Although in the main this may be the CYP and the therapist, at times parents or friends or significant others could be involved in the therapy as a co-therapist to help the CYP at home and strengthen the support in challenging some of their difficulties. CBT can also be offered in a group setting for some difficulties. CBT is generally in the here and now, although previous experiences are considered in how they may have impacted on the presenting problem. CBT bases itself on empirical evidence, meaning that theories and practice of CBT are evaluated as much as possible to demonstrate its scientific value and effectiveness (Westbrook et al. 2011). CBT does involve the use of Routine Outcome Measures (ROMs) to help identify progress and the helpfulness of CBT and also help understand the development and maintenance of the problem (Hawton et al. 1989). The Child Outcome Research Consortium (CORC) is a national website where you can access free ROMs and other useful information to use in your practice (https://www.corc.uk.net/) (CORC 2019a, b). CBT would deem the patient as the expert in their own life and see the therapist as bringing expertise to equip the patient with understanding, new experiences and strategies to manage and treat the problem and to support the patient in becoming their own therapist (Westbrook et al. 2011).

It is expected that every CBT session has a collaboratively developed agenda by the CYP and the therapist that will be completed throughout the session. One of the final agenda items will include a 'homework task', or 'activities for home'. Activities for home is a useful phrase if the CYP struggles with the concept of homework; and helps move it away from the school structure. The homework or activities for home is an essential part of the CBT model and is used to inform the subsequent session (Hawton et al. 1989). Without the homework or activities for home being completed, it will be very difficult to move forward with CBT and outcomes are significantly poorer (Kazantzis et al. 2000). It is helpful to describe CBT as offering 10% of the work in the session and 90% completed at home; this emphasises the importance of completing the home tasks but also helps encourage change outside the session where the problem has been developed and therfore will be best treated. Therefore, a CYP who is not willing to complete activites for home is unlikely to be suitable for CBT.

All of the aspects of CBT as detailed above should be initially discussed in a CBT suitability assessment with the CYP. A suitability assessment allows the CYP to socialise to the model of CBT and also offers the therapist time to assess motivation and whether the CYP wants to work within a CBT structure (Roos and Wearden 2009). It is really important to ensure that the therapy is the right fit for the CYP. The incorrect choice of therapy will impact on overall outcome and engagement.

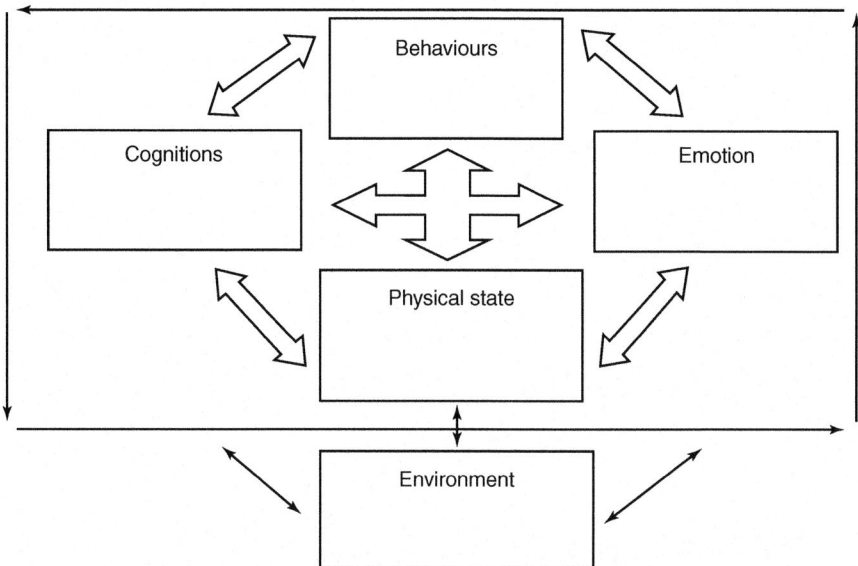

Fig. 9.2 5 systems model for CBT (Adapted from Padesky and Mooney 1990)

A basic and useful model or formulation used within CBT is that similar to Padesky and Mooney (1990), which captures the problem in diagrammatic form (see Fig. 9.2). Although this model was developed for CBT, it can be helpful in any assessment. The model demonstrates the relationship between behaviours, cognitions (thoughts), emotions and physiology, indicating that all of these areas have an effect on each other, as demonstrated earlier in the fear of a spider example. Throughout an assessment the therapist would use socratic dialogue to elicit the information needed to fully complete the model (Padesky 1993).

Once an understanding of the problem has been ascertained, the therapist and the CYP will decide together how to best treat the presenting problem. Treatment in CBT will aim to reduce the symptoms identified in the four systems of the model (behaviours, cognitions, emotion and physical state). This will, in turn, reduce the symptoms in another system. The therapist may start with the thought about 'the spider is going to get me' and develop a treatment strategy collaboratively with the CYP that targets this aspect. The treatment would help the CYP find new information to think differently about spider getting them, which will subsequently change the behaviours associated with that thought. Treatment in CBT has a wide variety of tools to use including psychoeducation, behavioural experiments, graded exposure, systematic desensitisation, in-vivo work, information collecting, fact finding and cognitive challenges (Bennett-Levy et al. 2004; Hawton et al. 1989; Westbrook et al. 2011). The determinant of treatment being successful is by the achieving of their goal-based outcomes (GBOs), which are set at the beginning of therapy (CORC 2019a, b).

Learning Point Summary
- CBT is a structured approach to therapy; the model will not suit CYPs who do not want to work in between sessions and do not want to challenge their difficulties.
- CBT is very collaborative and holds the collaboration as central to its philosophy, the therapist and CYP are equal in the therapeutic relationship.
- CBT is not just about changing thoughts and CYPs should not be referred for this alone.
- It is a short-term evidence-based treatment for a range of mental health difficulties.
- CBT works to an agenda and goal-based outcomes and uses ROMS throughout its process.
- CBT with CYP is systemically driven and differs from adult CBT.
- CBT with CYP can be creative and fun.

9.3.2   Psychodynamic Therapy

The development of psychoanalysis and psychoanalytic therapy has been discussed in this chapter. Psychodynamic therapy philosophy has developed from a range of theories including psychoanalytical, neuroscientific, attachment and developmental theory (Hobson 2015; Luyten et al. 2015; Berzoff et al. 2008).

Psychodynamic theory shares some core tenets with psychoanalytical theory in having equal focus on relationships. The focal points are on the relationship between the CYP and therapist, and the relationship between the CYP and his or her external world (Psychology Today 2019). Psychodynamic therapy usually involves a therapist and CYP being seen individually. It uses the knowledge of previous painful experiences, relationships and events to support the CYP in developing new patterns within relationships and subsequently finding ways to understand emotional experiences. This is done through exploring, clarifying and interpreting events with the CYP through a set of evidence-based interventions (Summers and Barber 2010). Psychodynamic therapy is evidence-based for depression and more recently eating disorders in current NICE guidance (2019).

Two key components within psychodynamic therapy are the considerations about transference and countertransference (Summers and Barber 2010). Both of these phenomena are embedded in the relationships that psychoanalytical and psychodynamic therapy study. Object relational theory helps the therapist to understand how the CYP is able to displace previous emotions and attitudes from their previous relationships, events and experiences to a substitute form or object, which is known as transference (Colman 2003; Brown 1964). Transference can be described in an example of a CYP having an anxious and excessively worried parent that has been overprotective toward the CYP throughout their childhood, which has prevented the CYP from taking many risks and subsequently inhibited developing independence in line with their peers. This relationship with the parent [the object] will be unconsciously replayed throughout the CYP's current and future relationships. By the therapist gaining some understanding of this process, this will enable the therapist to work with the CYP in developing new pathways in relationships without the object being played out (Sanfeliú and Walters 2014).

Countertransference is embedded within the relationship between the therapist and the CYP and the CYP's transference. The therapist's unconsciousness will replay in the therapeutic relationship with the CYP, similarly as in transference from parent to child (Colman 2003). The objects in transference and countertransference have considerable impact on the personal values and assumptions of the therapist and the CYP. It is important for both the therapist and the CYP to explore these and have some understanding of how these are impacting on therapy. Psychodynamic theorists argue that transference provokes a countertransference (King and O'Brien 2011); an example of this may be that a CYP who is working with the therapist is not engaging well in the process despite the therapist's best efforts. The therapist may start to feel that they are not confident in working with this particular CYP or their difficulty. The therapist becomes frustrated when meeting the CYP, holding feelings of inadequacy and feelings of being 'stuck' with the process. The therapist has either an opportunity to openly discuss their feelings with the CYP in an attempt to understand the countertransference to work through the difficulties or the therapist may infer from these feelings that the CYP is not motivated for therapy and ends the relationship. By the therapist having knowledge of transference and countertransference and being able to discuss this with the CYP, then therapy difficulties from transference and countertransference can be worked through (King and O'Brien 2011).

Learning Point Summary
- Psychodynamic therapy is a medium-term intervention that focuses on relationships.
- It is evidence-based for depression and eating disorders.
- Psychodynamic theory uses object relational theory to help understand relationships.
- Two key structures within psychodynamic theory are transference and countertransference.
- It is usually the CYP and the therapist that attend therapy and no other persons involved.

9.3.3 Systemic Family Therapy

The evolution of family therapy has been briefly discussed in this chapter in that it was developed formerly out of marriage counselling and extended its role to couples and then toward families. There have been many models of family therapy developed over the years including the Milan, strategic, structural and affective experiential models (Israelstam 1988). Systemic family therapy (SFT) particularly focuses on systems, relationships and dynamics that encompass families and their wider systems. SFT works from a strengths-based model to explore and make useful changes within the systems and the relationships to treat the difficulties (Association for Family Therapy 2019). SFT is currently evidence-based for eating disorders, anti-social behaviour and conduct disorder, bipolar disorder, depression and schizophrenia (NICE 2019).

SFT's model of therapy allows for many variations of family groupings to be involved in the therapy at different points depending on the need and difficulties of the family having therapy. At times all family members (those integrally related to the difficulty) may take part; in other sessions there may be two or three people from the family and at times there could be just one person. SFT also reaches the wider system outside the family if it is felt important to do so (Stratton 2016). SFT is also undertaken in groups in a multi-family therapy (MFT) session; this is particularly evidence-based for working with eating disorder difficulties. MFT is where there are usually six to eight families working in one session with a number of therapists and they will endeavour to develop healthy family relationships and routines and support families in working together to achieve this (Dawson et al. 2018).

SFT reflecting teams observe the therapy that the family is having. A reflecting team is not compulsory but can be useful in complex situations or where the therapist may have difficulty in keeping neutral to the content of the discussion. It is important for the therapist to not align to any one member of the family and in order to do this must have a distinct understanding of one's own values and assumptions (Totsuka 2014). The reflecting team observes the therapy this may be visually or audibly and will intermittently, when needed, discuss their observations of the therapy session and discuss what they perceive is happening in therapy. The reflecting team keeps separate from the therapist and family and there is not any conversation between the two parties. The family will hear these discussions and the outcomes of the discussion will be included in the ongoing therapy (Andersen 1987). Consent is always needed from every attending member of the family for the reflecting team to be observing; for more information on gaining consent see Chap. 11.

SFT theorists when working with CYP would advocate for therapists to work more creatively in order to better understand the CYP and make the experience more meaningful, similarly as in CBT. SFT prides itself on ensuring inclusivity in working in a family orientated approach and the importance of the CYP being heard within it. SFT places equal value to all perspectives and therapists position themselves in being neutral to all the family and its dynamics that span the system. The therapist continually works with self and self-reflexivity in maintaining the neutrality. The therapist focuses on maintaining neutrality during supervision and within the reflecting teams (Andersen 1987; Dallos and Draper 2010).

SFT uses three principles of hypothesising, neutrality and circularity to gain information and create the space. Hypothesising is about making sense of the information that is available, circularity in relation to maintain the hypotheses but also to consider new possibilities of making sense of the information and neutrality is about the therapist remaining neutral and equally valuing each member of the family and its wider systems (Brown 2010).

Learning Point Summary

- SFT is a family-based therapy that involves all necessary members of the family.
- It is a medium-term therapy.
- SFT is evidence-based for a number of mental health disorders.
- SFT is open to using ideas and theories from other models of psychotherapy.
- At times reflecting teams are part of the therapy.
- SFT holds the therapist in being neutral and valuing all family members as equal.
- The therapist has to use self and reflexive use of self to maintain neutrality.

9.3.4   Other Therapies Used in CAMHS

Some other widely used therapies in CAMHS are Dialectical Behavioural Therapy (DBT) which was developed by Marsha Linehan (1993). Linehan combines traditional CBT strategies with more eastern philosophies, such as Zen practices. DBT requires the therapist to manage opposing forces and attempt to reconcile through synthesis, whilst offering acceptance to the patient throughout. Linehan describes the most opposing force as asking them patient to change whilst accepting the patient just as they are. These opposing forces are the dialectal attributes of the therapy (Ibid). DBT is a manualised, skills-based approach that is evidenced for adolescents aged 15 years or over that are self-harming or have emerging personality disorders (NICE 2009).

Eye Movement Desensitisation Reprocessing (EMDR) is an evidence-based therapy that uses eye movement to process trauma. One of the main attributes of the trauma focused therapy is that CYP do not have to talk or verbalise the trauma, they can just bring it to mind (Shapiro 2012). This is helpful when thinking about trauma work with CYP who don't want to discuss the trauma; however, some find talking through the trauma more helpful, so trauma focused CBT may be appropriate.

Interpersonal therapy (IPT) is an evidence-based therapy for depression. IPT considers the interpersonal contexts and relationships around the patient to make sense of the depression (Interpersonal Psychotherapy UK (IPTUK) 2019).

9.4   Some Common Themes Across Therapies

9.4.1   Communication

Communication is one of the key considerations when working with CYP. It is important to remember that the way that you construct language and understand as adult will be very different from that of a CYP. As adults we make a number of assumptions about CYP and parents in that we speak in words that they understand. This is frequently not the case and holding these assumptions can cause significant difficulties and misunderstandings in therapy. The use of jargon and medical language should be avoided at all times, as should the use of long words. Unfortunately, the position of power remains with the therapist, no matter how the therapist or nurse attempts to shift the power and become more collaborative. This means that despite best efforts of ensuring the CYP understands what is being said, the CYP may state that they understand, even when they don't. Certainly, using more pictorial or diagrammatic ways of communicating can help the CYP or parent understand more easily. There is further information about facilitating aspects of engagement in relation to consent in Chap. 11.

Non-verbal communication is also extremely important throughout therapy. Gerard Egan refers to the acronym SOLER which stands for:

Squarely—Facing the CYP squarely to visually demonstrate concentrating on the CYP.
Open—Create an open posture to demonstrate welcoming talking to the CYPs.
Lean—Toward the CYP to demonstrate closeness and interest.
Eye Contact—Should be helpfully maintained to demonstrate attentiveness.
Relax—To keep a calm environment to support the CYP in being at ease (Egan 2014:59).

In therapy, non-verbal communication is considered as important as what the therapist or CYP is verbally communicating. The communication that is being seen non-verbally can help understanding but can also hinder the therapy if not addressed. It is important for the therapist to be self-aware what they are communicating non-verbally and ensure that their non-verbal communication is matching their verbal communication. When there is a mismatch in this, this can cause confusion for the CYP (Egan 2014; Foley and Gentile 2010). Many of these skills are learned as part of the nurse training curriculum and are easily transferable to working therapeutically with children.

9.4.2   The Therapeutic Relationship (TR)

The therapeutic relationship is well documented to be an extremely important part of therapy, with the quality of the relationship being evidenced as a good predictor of outcome (Orlinsky et al. 1994). The TR is regarded slightly differently within the different domains of therapy, but all consider TR as significantly important (Dallos and Draper 2010; Summers and Barber 2010; Westbrook et al. 2011). The TR can be thought of as the concept that holds the relationship between the therapist and the CYP. This may be thought of slightly differently between therapies; however, the TR is seen as a vehicle for which therapy is conveyed through, but also holds the relationship and the associated attributes within it; some examples of these attributes are trust, respect, humour, attachment, empathy, expectation and safety (Gilbert and Leahy 2007); in essence, it is the therapeutic glue that holds the therapist and CYP in place and enables the therapy to progress. Ruptures in the TR are well-known phenomena and can be very difficult to resolve if not caught early. These signs can be picked up through non-verbal communication or lack of engagement. By using the relationship to work through these ruptures at an early point will be beneficial in re-engaging and motivating the CYP to continue progressing through therapy (Watson and Greenberg 2000). Nurses will have much experience in developing the TR; however, the importance of it may have not been envisaged. Developing the TR skills further to support therapeutic intervention will be within the nurse's ability.

9.5 Supervision

Supervision is one of the key structures throughout psychotherapy. Supervision is used to aid learning and to help therapists to review and explore difficulties that have developed in therapy. This may be due to a difficult event, a learning need of the therapist or to ensure fidelity to the specific model of therapy (Gilbert and Evans 2000). Supervision should be seen as a facilitative action that bases itself in curiosity and a learning environment. Supervision is important when undertaking any clinical activity within CAMHS and should be used effectively by the nurse. This includes the supervisee in being prepared and using supervision well. Supervision is a good space to reflect on personal values and assumptions about the therapist and how this may be impacting on therapy itself; this will support personal and professional growth of the supervisee.

9.6 Routine Outcome Measures (ROMs)

ROMs are used variably throughout therapy. The CYP-IAPT data set uses a wide range of ROMs and for those therapies that are taught within the CYP-IAPT programme, there is an expectation to use those ROMs from the data set (NHSE 2018a). Many therapies align themselves to the use of goals in order to offer a common end point of therapy (Dallos and Draper 2010; Summers and Barber 2010; Westbrook et al. 2011). ROMs have the ability to measure many different aspects of therapy. These can be the progress of the CYP in relation to symptom reduction and global functioning. ROMs can also measure some aspects of the therapeutic alliance on a session by session basis (CORC 2019a, b) and can measure specific aspects of the therapeutic relationship such as empathy (Burns and Auerback 1996). Using ROMs clinically effectively is an important skill for the nurse to develop. The use of ROMs has been demonstrated to be useful way of measuring progress and enables the nurse to adapt therapeutic intervention from the feedback from the ROMs to ensure optimum use of the therapy itself.

Learning Point Summary
- There are many commonalities that cross all psychotherapies.
- Being aware of personal values and assumptions are key in all aspects of therapy.
- Supervision is a significant part of therapy that needs to be used effectively.
- ROMs can be used across the spectrum of therapy and is expected as part of the CYP-IAPT strategy.
- Fundamental verbal and non-verbal communication skills are paramount in developing the therapeutic relationship and maintaining therapy.
- Nurses are equipped with many of the skills needed to develop and maintain therapy and the therapeutic relationship.

This chapter has given an overview of some of the main therapies used within CAMHS and detailed some of key skills needed in order to develop the therapeutic relationship and progress with therapy. Many of the nurse skills acquired through training will be transferable in the therapeutic arena. Nurses are in prime position to employ and develop their nursing skills in using evidence-based therapeutic interventions. The nurse is able to use transferable skills in an effective and meaningful way to offer intervention throughout psychotherapy models when accessing quality supervision and guidance.

Acknowledgements Acknowledgement to Leah Benson RMN and Mark Sumpter RMN for the support and guidance in producing this chapter.

References

Andersen T (1987) The reflecting team: dialogue and meta-dialogue in clinical work. Fam Pract 26:415–428

Association for Family Therapy (2019) What is family therapy [online]. http://www.aft.org.uk/consider/view/family-therapy.html. Accessed 31 Jan 2019

Beck AT (1967) Depression: the causes and treatment. University of Pennsylvania Press, Philadelphia

Bennett-Levy J, Butler G, Fennell M, Hackman A, Mueller M, Westbrook D (2004) Oxford guide to behavioural experiments in cognitive therapy. Oxford University press, Oxford

Berzoff J, Flanagan LM, Hertz P (eds) (2008) Psychodynamic clinical theory and psychopathology in contemporary multi-cultural contexts, 2nd edn. Jason Aronson, Plymouth

Brown JAC (1964) Freud and the post-Freudians. Penguin books, Middlesex

Brown JM (2010) The Milan principles of hypothesising circularity and neutrality in dialogical family therapy: extinction, evolution, eviction… or emergence? Aust N Z J Fam Ther 31(3):248–265

Burns DD, Auerback A (1996) Therapeutic empathy in cognitive behaviour therapy: does it make a difference? In: Salkovskis PM (ed) Frontiers of cognitive therapy. Guilford Press, New York, pp 135–164

Byng-Hall J (1982) Dysfunctions of feeling: experiential life of the family. In: Bentovim A, Barnes GG, Cooklin A (eds) Family therapy: complementary frameworks of theory and practice, vol 1. Academic Press, London, pp 59–78

Child and Adolescent Mental Health Services (2008) Children and young people in mind: the final report of the national CAMHS review (the final report) [online]. http://webarchive.nationalar-

chives.gov.uk/20081230004520/publications.dcsf.gov.uk/eorderingdownload/camhs-review.
pdf. Accessed 20 Dec 2018

Colman AM (2003) Oxford dictionary of psychology. Oxford University Press, Oxford

CORC (2019a) Child Outcomes Research Consortium [online]. https://www.corc.uk.net/.
Accessed 12 Jan 2019

CORC (2019b) Goal based outcomes [online]. https://www.corc.uk.net/outcome-experience-mea-
sures/goal-based-outcomes/. Accessed 12 Jan 2019

Dallos R, Draper R (2010) An introduction into family therapy. Systemic theory and practice, 3rd
edn. Open University Press, Berkshire

Dendy WC (1853) Pscyhe: a discourse on the birth and pilgrimage of thought. Longmans, Browns,
Green & Longmans, London

Dawson L, Baudinet J, Tay E, Wallis A (2018) Creating community—the introduction of multi-
family therapy for eating disorders in Australia. Aust N Z J Fam Ther 39:283–293

Department of Health & NHS England (2015) Future in mind. Crown Copyright, London

DHSC & DE (2018) Transforming children and young people's mental health provision: a green
paper and next steps [online]. https://assets.publishing.service.gov.uk/government/uploads/
system/uploads/attachment_data/file/728892/government-response-to-consultation-on-trans-
forming-children-and-young-peoples-mental-health.pdf. Accessed 5 Jan 2018

Dubois P (1905) The psychic treatment of nervous disorders: the psychoneuroses and their moral
treatment. In: Jelliffe SE (Trans), White WA (Trans). Funk & Wagnalls, New York

Egan G (2014) The skilled helper: a client centred approach. Cengage Learning EMEA,
Hampshire

Ellis A (1962) Reason and emotion in psychotherapy. Stuart Lyle, New York

Evrard R, Pratte EA, Cardeña E (2018) Pierre Janet and the enchanted boundary of psychical
research. Hist Psychol 21(2):100–125

Foley GN, Gentile JP (2010) Non-verbal communication in psychotherapy. Psychiatry (Edgmont)
7(6):38–44

Gilbert P, Leahy RL (eds) (2007) The therapeutic relationship in the cognitive behavioral psychotherapies. Routledge/Taylor & Francis Group, New York

Gilbert MC, Evans K (2000) Psychotherapy supervision: an integrative relational approach to psychotherapy supervision. Open University Press, Buckingham

Greene BL, Solomon AP (1963) Marital disharmony: concurrent psychoanalytic therapy of
husband and wife by the same psychiatrist. The triangular transference transactions. Am J
Psychother 17:443–450

Haley J (1962) Family experiments: a new type of experiment. Fam Process 1:265–291

Hawton K, Salkovskis PM, Kirk J, Clark DM (eds) (1989) Cognitive behavioural therapy for psychiatric problems. A practical guide. Oxford University Press, Oxford

Hayes ST, Hofmann SG (2017) The third wave of cognitive behavioral therapy and the rise of
process-based care. World Psychiatry 16(3):245–246

Hobson A (2015) Psychodynamic neurology: dreams, consciousness, and virtual reality. Taylor
and Francis Group, London

Howells J (ed) (1971) Theory and practice of family psychiatry. Brunner/Mazel, New York

IPTUK (2019) Interpersonal psychotherapy UK network [online]. https://www.iptuk.net/.
Accessed 12 Jan 2012

Israelstam K (1988) Contrasting four major family therapy paradigms: implications for family
therapy training. J Fam Ther 101:179–196

Jung C (1959) The archetypes and the collective unconscious. Bollingen Foundation, New York

Kaslow FW (2000) History of family therapy. J Fam Psychother 11(4):1–35

Kazantzis N, Deane FP, Ronan KR (2000) Homework assignments in cognitive and Behavioral
therapy: a meta-analysis. Clin Psychol Sci Prac 7:189–202

King R, O'Brien T (2011) Transference and countertransference: opportunities and risks as
two technical constructs migrate beyond their psychoanalytic homeland. Psychother Aust
17(4):12–17

Klein M (1960) The psychoanalyses of children [online]. https://archive.org/details/psychoanaly-
sisof007950mbp/page/n7. Accessed 6 Jan 2019

Linehan M (1993) Skills training manual for treating borderline personality disorder. Guilford Press, New York

Luyten P, Mayes LC, Fonagy P, Target M, Blatt SJ (eds) (2015) Handbook of psychodynamic approaches to psychopathology. Guilford Press, London

Mills JA (1998) Control: a history of behavioural psychology. New York University Press, London

NHSE (2018a) CYP-IAPT programme [online]. https://www.england.nhs.uk/mental-health/cyp/iapt/. Accessed 20 Dec 2018

NHSE (2018b) Adult improving access to psychological therapies programme [online]. https://www.england.nhs.uk/mental-health/adults/iapt/. Accessed 20 Dec 2018

NICE (2009) NICE guidance CG78: borderline personality disorder: recognition and management [online]. https://www.nice.org.uk/guidance/cg78. Accessed 12 Jan 2019

NICE (2019) National Institute for Health and Care Excellence [online]. https://www.nice.org.uk/. Accessed 6 Jan 2019

Orlinsky D, Grawe K, Parkes B (1994) Process and outcome in psychotherapy. In: Bergin AE, Garfield SL (eds) Handbook of psychotherapy and behavior change. Wiley, Oxford, pp 270–376

Padesky CA (1993) Socratic questioning: changing minds or guided discovery? European Congress of Behavioural and Cognitive Therapies, London, September 1994

Padesky CA, Mooney KA (1990) Presenting the cognitive model to clients. Int Cognit Ther Newsl 6:13–14

Psychology Today (2019) Psychodynamic therapy [online]. https://www.psychologytoday.com/gb/therapy-types/psychodynamic-therapy. Accessed 29 Jan 2019

Robertson D (2010) The philosophy of cognitive-behavioural therapy (CBT). Stoic philosophy as rational and cognitive psychotherapy. Karnac Books Ltd., London

Roos J, Wearden A (2009) What do we mean by "socialization to the model"? A Delphi study. Behav Cogn Psychother 37(3):341–345

Rubovits-Seitz PFD (2014) Kohut's Freudian vision. Routledge, London

Sanfeliú I, Walters K (2014) Karl Abraham: the birth of object relations theory (trans: Sanfeliú I, Walters K). Karnac Books Ltd., London

Shapiro F (2012) Getting past your past. Take control of your life with self-help techniques from EMDR therapy. Rodale Books, New York

Skynner R (1976) Systems of family and marital psychotherapy. Brunner/Maze, New York

Solms M, Saling M (1986) On psychoanalysis and neuroscience: Freud's attitude to the localizationist tradition. Int J Psychoanal 67(4):397–416

Steimer T (2002) The biology of fear and anxiety related behaviours. Dialogues Clin Neurosci 4(3):231–249

Stratton P (2016) The evidence base of family therapy and systemic practice. Association for Family Therapy, Warrington

Summers RF, Barber JP (2010) Psychodynamic therapy: a guide to evidenced based practice. Guilford press, New York

Totsuka Y (2014) Which aspects of social GGRRAAACCEEESSS grab you most?' The social GGRRAAACCEEESSS exercise for a supervision group to promote therapists' self-reflexivity. J Fam Ther 36(1):86–106

Wallace ER, Gach J (eds) (2008) History of psychiatry and medical psychology. Springer, New York

Watson JC, Greenberg LS (2000) Alliance rupture and repairs in experiential therapy. J Clin Psychol 56(2):175–188

Westbrook D, Kennerley H, Kirk J (2011) An introduction to cognitive behavioural therapy: skills and applications. Sage, London

Wolpe J (1969) The practice of behavioral therapy. Pergamon Press, Ltd., New York

Wolpert M, Harris R, Jones M, Hodges S, Fuggle P, James R, Weiner A, Mckenna C, Law D, Fonagy P (2014) THRIVE. The AFC-Tavistock model for CAMHS [online]. https://www.gmecscn.nhs.uk/attachments/article/196/Thrive%20model%20for%20CAMHS.pdf. Accessed 4 Jan 2019

Chapter 10
CAMHS Self-Harm Teams and Crisis/Liaison Teams; What CAMH Nurses Bring to the Acute Moments in Young People's Lives

Marie Armstrong

10.1   Introduction

This chapter focuses on one of the places where young people who self-harm are in contact with services, the general hospital. This includes their experience in the Emergency Department and on hospital wards—usually paediatric wards where young people under the age of 16 are admitted overnight, as recommended by NICE guidelines (NICE 2004).

Most self-harm hospital attendances are due to having taken an overdose, but also include young people who have cut themselves, have harmed themselves in other ways or are having suicidal thoughts. Most young people come to hospital because they are in a 'crisis' and require urgent physical and/or mental health assessment or intervention. For some however, it may feel like an unwanted but necessary attendance, perhaps because they need physical treatment when they have attended before and already have a plan in place, rather than them feeling they are in crisis. Recent guidance (NCCMH 2016) has set out exceptions—circumstances in which a divergence can occur with young people under 16 not being admitted to hospital.

Just as not all young people attending hospital for self-harm may consider themselves to be in crisis, many young people are self-harming in the community some of whom are 'in crisis' but not accessing appropriate services. The skills discussed in this chapter are transferable to different contexts where the crisis may occur. Self-harm should never be ignored. Holly reflects how she needed help for a long time before things escalated with her ending up in hospital and finally getting an assessment and the help she needed.

M. Armstrong (✉)
Hopewood, Nottinghamshire Healthcare NHS Foundation Trust, Nottingham, UK
e-mail: Marie.Armstrong@nottshc.nhs.uk

© Springer Nature Switzerland AG 2020   155
L. Baldwin (ed.), *Nursing Skills for Children and Young People's Mental Health*,
https://doi.org/10.1007/978-3-030-18679-1_10

At school I did PE for 3 years whilst self-harming almost every day; my cuts/scars were visible when in shorts and a polo shirt. During this time not one teacher asked me if I was okay or if I needed help. (Holly—now aged 25)

The help young people need will vary greatly depending on many factors, so their needs should be matched appropriately across a self-harm care pathway from universal to highly specialist services—an example of which is enclosed in Fig. 10.1.

Different CAMHS across the UK have different structures and teams, but often their services include CAMHS self-harm teams or CAMHS crisis/liaison teams whose role is to undertake urgent hospital/community assessments. The majority of staff in these teams are mental health nurses; this chapter focuses on the nursing skills, sometimes explicit, more often subtle and notoriously difficult to articulate that are used in this context to provide high quality risk and needs assessments to young people who self-harm and present in crisis.

10.2   Definition of Crisis

'A mental health crisis is a situation which the child, young person, family member, carer or any other person believes requires an immediate response, assistance and/ or care from a mental health service, including where there is significant intent or risk of harm to themselves or others. A mental health crisis can have a wide range of underlying causes, diagnoses and triggers, some of which may be longstanding, but which essentially culminate in a deterioration of an individual's mental state to the point at which they require an immediate response from mental health services' (NCCMH 2016).

In practice, different services have different ideas about what constitutes a crisis—CAMHS teams are set up for managing mental health crisis with a remit of where appropriate and safe to do so, preventing admission of young people to in-patient psychiatric adolescent units. Implicit in this is the idea that they support young people who otherwise would meet the criteria for admission. Many young people who experience a crisis do not have mental illness and would not meet the criteria threshold for admission and therefore may not be offered a service by mental health crisis teams.

It is acknowledged that underlying reasons and contributing factors to the crisis are often complex and require multi-agency working addressing social, health, educational and other needs. In practice, there is sometimes a risk that young people can fall between gaps in service provision, so nurses in CAMHS crisis teams work holistically, using their advocacy skills, supporting young people to gain access to the services required to meet their needs. In these situations, CAMH nurses utilise their communication skills, clarifying the remit of teams and services and signposting to other organisations as needed.

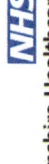

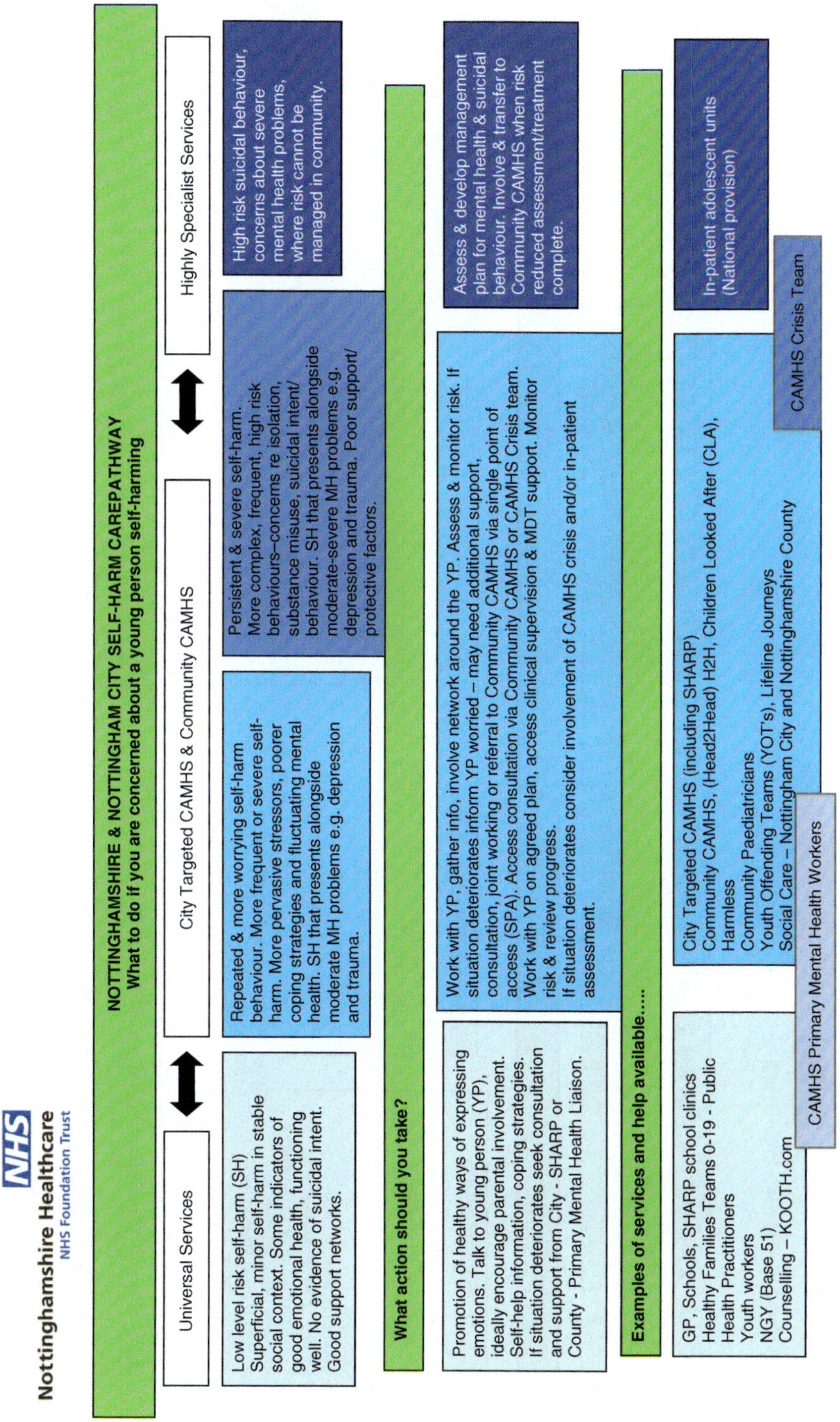

Fig. 10.1 Notts Healthcare NHSFT Self-harm pathways (used with kind permission)

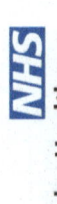

NHS

Nottinghamshire Healthcare
NHS Foundation Trust

Monitor & document concerns, seek appropriate supervision and involvement of line manager.
IN THE CASE OF A MEDICAL EMERGENCY REFER YOUNG PERSON TO THEIR GP OR HOSPITAL EMERGENCY DEPARTMENT IMMEDIATELY
YP under 16 who attend emergency department for self-harm will usually be admitted & assessed following day or may be assessed same day by
CAMHS Crisis Team. 16 & 17 year olds may be assessed by Adult Mental Health Services and referred to Targeted/community CAMHS for follow-up.
IN THE CASE OF A MENTAL HEALTH EMERGENCY CONTACT CAMHS CRISIS TEAM VIA SPA ON 8542299 (M-F) OR 8440560 (M-F 8-10 & S-S 10-6)

Examples of interventions……

RANGE OF INTERVENTIONS

Assessment and management of
suicidal risk & serious self-harm
Assessment & treatment of mental
illness

Urgent assessment &
intervention in response to
immediate risk.
Home treatment

RANGE OF INTERVENTIONS

Risk & needs assessment/formulation
Mental health assessments – where appropriate diagnosis
Individual psychotherapy, Systemic/Family Therapy, CBT, DBT, EMDR, group
work, support for parents
Consultation to CAMHS staff
Prescribing/medication review

Consultation to universal services
& teaching

RANGE OF INTERVENTIONS

Assessment
Family work/ individual work
Counselling
Mentoring
Group work
Psycho-education
Resilience building, self-esteem
Early Help Assessment Framework
– self-harm risk reduction
NVR (Non-Violent Resistance)
Liaison/signposting

THIS CAREPATHWAY IS FOR USE IN CONJUNCTION WITH NOTTINGHAMSHIRE & NOTTINGHAM CITY PRACTICE
GUIDANCE ON CHILDREN & YOUNG PEOPLE WHO SELF-HARM.

M Armstrong: Nurse Consultant CAMHS – Self-harm October 2018

Fig. 10.1 (continued)

10.3 Use of Crisis Point

There are many reasons why self-harm gets to a crisis point for young people; this may partly depend on whether it is the first time they have self-harmed or if they have self-harmed before. The first time may present as a crisis point in itself, or for someone who has self-harmed many times before, if they self-harm in a more serious way, e.g. cut themselves more deeply or on a different part of their body, or if their motivation and intent is different than previously, e.g. they feel they cannot take anymore and want to end their life. Sometimes things get to a crisis point very quickly and on other occasions there is a gradual descent into crisis. We should never underestimate the magnitude of what it may be like for young people and parents to access help, especially in a crisis, we need to use our skills of self-reflection to be curious and wonder what it is like to be in each of their 'particular shoes'.

It is often asked why increasing numbers of young people are self-harming; contributing factors appear to be academic pressures, physical health conditions, bullying, social isolation and social media. Overall the huge amount of pressures that young people feel to fit in, be accepted and 'get it right' can feel overwhelming and with social media these pressures are 24/7 with no rest. The CAMH nurse uses their skills to understand this context, and validate their experience in the young person's world.

They may feel embarrassed, ashamed, guilty and/or scarred—emotions that are difficult to deal with and can result in internal stigma—the young person judging and blaming themselves. They may also experience or anticipate external stigma, discussed further on in this chapter, preventing them from sharing and reaching out for help.

In view of this, young people often try to sort out problems themselves, sometimes with the help of friends who young people tell us are often the first people to know about their self-harm. Inevitably, for some young people things escalate, some of the most common expressions that young people share with CAMH nurses when they reach crisis point are:

I thought I could manage but it all got too much,

I never thought I would do this

Yesterday was the worst day ever

I just felt I couldn't go on like that anymore, I just couldn't bear it

Sometimes, the shock and experience of reaching 'rock bottom', i.e. crisis point, together with a high quality risk and needs assessment by the CAMH nurse, where the young person feels listened to and validated, can result in realisation and produce hope and motivation for positive change.

All of this is in the context of adolescent development, a time when young people are still developing their problem-solving skills, they do not have the benefit of vast life experience helping them through complex, painful, social situations. Some more than others may have a tendency to be impulsive, experience rapid mood changes and find it hard to tolerate high levels of distress.

Sometimes young people and parents tell us they have been trying to access help for some time prior to the situation reaching a crisis point and they have not felt listened to, taken seriously or referred to services they feel could help.

Once a young person is in crisis, if they have not received a service before, they can feel a sense of relief and use the opportunity to off-load the difficulties they have been experiencing. If on the other hand they are already known to CAMHS, and have a lead professional and agreed plan, they sometimes find it difficult talking to a different person who they may not have met before, so they can feel frustrated feeling they are 'going over' things that other people already know to someone they may not see again.

The CAMH nurse aims to meet the needs of all young people presenting in many different circumstances. They need to use their skills to judge the amount of information needed from a young person, whether to just focus on the immediate presentation, risk and needs or to build up a much bigger narrative, placing the immediate risks and needs in greater context.

What is absolutely critical is that it is taken seriously and without judgement. Contributing to this is the importance of the skill of use of language used by the CAMH nurse. NICE (2004) have challenged the use of pejorative terms such as 'deliberate' and 'commit'—but the casual, unthoughtful use of other language can unintentionally undermine and make young people feel worthless.

As Holly explains:
Whilst the word 'superficial' might be a clinical term, using it in front of someone who has self-harmed, or describing someone's self-harm as superficial when speaking to them, can lead to their self-harm getting even worse. As someone with a long history of self-harm, that word has lead to me feeling my self-harm wasn't good enough, that it was pathetic and that I was too. It has caused me to self-harm in a more destructive way, needing stitches. The word superficial may seem harmless, but it can be dangerous.

10.4   The Role and Key Skills of CAMH Nurses

The role and skills of mental health nurses are well documented (Callaghan et al. 2009; Callaghan and Gamble 2015) but much less is written about mental health nursing in CAMHS; in fact, concern has been raised about the impact of this lack of professional identity (Baldwin 2008). The paucity of empirical evidence does however leave an opportunity to describe a wealth of practice-based evidence—to create a written record of the key skills used by CAMH nurses day in day out in their work, in this chapter with young people who self-harm in crisis.

Two significant differences between CAMH nurses and other mental health nurses is their role in working with children and young people aged 0–18, therefore spanning a huge developmental range and working with them in the context of their families; parents and siblings. The CAMH nurse uses their skills to adapt to the young person's developmental stage and abilities and holds in mind and engages with where appropriate all members of the family.

The recent development of a competence framework for self-harm and suicide prevention in children and young people recommends skills and knowledge for professionals across a broad range of backgrounds and experiences (NCCMH 2018). The skills described in this chapter may not be exclusive to CAMH nurses but they are central to, and are the essence of CAMH nursing.

10.5 Care

The use of the term care or caring is synonymous with that of mental health nursing and being a mental health nurse. It immediately sets the scene that the mental health nursing role is about the relationship the nurse has with the 'patient', their values and beliefs, attitude towards them and the skills of providing a safe, respectful space from which help can be given. Peplau (1952) formed the basis of this is her theoretical model from which mental health nursing has continued to develop.

10.6 Therapeutic Relationship

Following on from Peplau (1952), 'Decades of empirical research have consistently linked the quality of the alliance between therapist and client with therapy outcome, independent of the type of therapy' (Horvath 2001).

In child and adolescent mental health nursing, the therapeutic relationship that is formed, not only between the nurse and the young person, but also where appropriate with the parents/family is critical both for assessment and on-going work/intervention. This means the skills of the CAMH nurse go beyond the technical ability to apply a theory/model/knowledge, to the skills of relational competence. The relationship is not the background in which change occurs but central to enabling change to occur, using the skills of analysing the interpersonal process as it emerges (Fruggeri 2012).

Thus the ability to use the skills of reflecting in and on action described in Schon's seminal work is essential (Schön 1983). Reflecting in action is particularly critical in this context, not only due to the need to react to the crisis situation at the time it occurs, including decisions about discharge and safety planning, but in order to 'see', 'experience', and 'bear witness' to the therapeutic relationship that is developing.

Implicit in this is the CAMH nurse bringing 'themselves' to the relationship and therefore personal factors playing a key part. It therefore needs to be recognised that sometimes the relationship is not working, i.e. there is not a 'fit' and people don't 'click', it doesn't feel right together. This is important to recognise so, if appropriate, another worker can be found in a helpful, constructive way that will then enable to young person to form a relationship that will enable them to be helped. This may not be possible during the assessment process but it can be acknowledged and planned for future sessions/therapeutic work. This ability and use of skills to 'get alongside' young people is invaluable, to engage with them on their level, having a grounded, empathic 'human' connection.

10.7 Personal and Professional Boundaries

One of the things that seems to be very important to young people is the nurse's fine-tuned skills around personal and professional boundaries. Professional in the sense of trustworthy, reliable, excellent communication and interpersonal skills but equally young people tell us they want the nurse to be approachable, friendly, warm, use a sense of humour and be prepared to share appropriate personal experiences— enabling a human connection. The balance to this is maintaining clear professional boundaries, not over-disclosing personal information, not contacting people outside of a work context, not forming relationships that go beyond work in line with our professional code of conduct (NMC 2018). Holly described her positive experiences of the above as CAMH nurses being what she coined as 'professionally friendly'. Being skilled and comfortable in taking this position seems to be one of the factors that enables mental health nurses in CAMHS to excel in conducting risk and needs assessments and may be one of the reasons why they are the profession of choice in self-harm/crisis/liaison teams.

As well as the therapeutic relationship there are also some overarching philosophies and values critical to high quality nursing care, such as having a person-centred approach (Rogers 1951) which is still as relevant today as it was in the 1950s. More recently, we received a salient reminder of nursing values in the form of the six C's: Care, Compassion, Competence, Communication, Courage and Commitment (DH 2012).

These are particularly relevant when working with young people who self-harm as they report many examples of experiencing lack of compassion, feeling judged and struggling with both internal and external stigma.

'Felt stigma, internal stigma or self-stigmatization, refers to the shame and expectation of discrimination that prevents people from talking about their experiences and stops them seeking help. Enacted stigma, external stigma, discrimination, refers to the experience of unfair treatment by others. Felt stigma can be as damaging as enacted stigma since it leads to withdrawal and restriction of social support' (Gray 2002).

It is ironic that self-harm is often perceived negatively by others as 'attention seeking' when for many young people it is hidden and only when they experience the 'right' care and compassion do they use their courage to communicate and share with others. It is hoped, with NICE guidelines (2004) feeling necessary to emphasise and promote that people who self-harm should be treated with the same care and respect as others, that young people have since experienced improvements in this area.

10.8 Physical Environment

Whilst the physical environment is important for 'setting the scene and context', for helping to make people feel comfortable and more at ease to talk, we may have limited choices about the venue where we see young people, the space and décor of the room. In a hospital setting there may be medical equipment in some rooms and no windows in others; these constraints can be acknowledged as far from ideal by the nurses to the young person and family. Where options are available, making it young person friendly, e.g. therapeutic colours, displaying positive messages and quotes, pictures and relaxed soft furnishing all contributes to creating a therapeutic space or milieu.

Whatever the context and constraints, some things cannot be compromised; the need for a private, confidential space without interruptions is essential. All contact with young people would include an explanation of their rights to confidentiality and the limitations of this where there are concerns about significant harm.

10.9 Confidentiality

Nurses need to be skilled in understanding the difference between a right to confidentiality and a young person's wishes. For example, a discussion should always be had with the young person about what information they are happy to share with parents either themselves or via the nurse. It is an error to assume that a person doesn't want their parents to know anything, when they are often happy for information to be shared if certain information is withheld.

At times of stress, communication can be compromised resulting in young people inaccurately thinking their parents don't know they self-harm. Discussing the young persons' reasons for not sharing information is important as often it is because they don't want to upset their parent or parents, when parents may know already or prefer to know/be less upset that they know.

These are skilled and often delicate conversations that need to be had, and repeated as the therapeutic relationship and trust develops and the work progresses. Just because a young person had a view not to share in the first session does not mean that has not changed over time.

10.10 Risk and Needs Assessment

A risk and needs assessment is the process of using evidence-based knowledge to ask pertinent questions to gather information in order to holistically understand the self-harm in context of the young person, their family, community and world.

In order to have as much consistency as possible across professionals and teams, many services use locally devised risk and needs assessment forms to give standardisation to the questions asked and the information obtained. Such a form should be regularly updated using all available evidence as to the most pertinent information needed. Whist the form is helpful for consistency and as an aide-memoire, it is only as good as the skills of the person using it. The risk and needs assessment process involves using a wide range of high level skills identified in this chapter; these will determine what information the young person chooses to share and thus the accuracy and quality of the understanding.

This is different from a risk assessment tool, which attempts to score and categorise risk, which we are warned against using for reasons stated in the following podcast:

> We need to step away from this false notion, fallacy, that we can predict the future, we shouldn't use risk assessment tools to predict what will happen to someone—as they don't work. Positive predictive values of risk assessment tools are low—20% of people who went on to repeat were missed by instruments and less than 50% of people rated as high went on to repeat. Most people who die by suicide are assessed as low risk.
>
> Instead, simply ask the young person do they think they are likely to repeat self-harm. Focus on needs based assessment—do our best to address needs, e.g. mental health, relationships, finances, physical health problems. Talking, listening and understanding what's going on for them may reduce risk by up to 40%—positive experience of empathy and plugging people into the correct services.
>
> Kapur N https://www.youtube.com/watch?v=fpmSqTQNeHc

10.11   Mental Health Problems

Part of a risk and needs assessment will be to assess if there are any associated mental health problems. Self-harm is a behaviour; something young people do, usually in response to overwhelming distress and their inability at the time to find an alternative way of coping. Some young people who self-harm may also have mental health problems such as depression, anxiety, post-traumatic stress or have experienced insecure attachments and have difficulties with emotional regulation, distress tolerance and interpersonal relationships. CAMH nurses use their knowledge, experience and the skills they have developed pre and post registration to identify any presence of mental health problems. The mental health nurse's experience of working in in-patient settings provides an opportunity for developing many skills in identifying different mental health presentations, taking into account individual variation, having a lens for the different degrees of severity and risk and the skills in managing these presentations. Where mental health problems are identified, appropriate evidence-based interventions and treatments should be discussed and referrals made to services that can provide these interventions.

10.12 Motivation and Links Between Self-Harm and Attempted Suicide

Every assessment aims to try and understand the motivation for the self-harm, the young person's intent. The CAMH nurse uses all the skills in this chapter to ascertain as best they can the purpose of the self-harm from the young person's point of view. Sometimes this will seem clear, e.g. the young person feels certain the cutting was to try and feel better, creating physical pain to take away emotional pain. Alternatively they may be clear they wanted to end their life, feeling they couldn't go on any longer. On other occasions, the young person may describe feeling uncertain, say they were not thinking or they did not care what happened, expressing ambivalence, saying part of them wanted to die and part of them did not.

Follow-up/interventions/therapy and safety plans will need to be different according to the different individual's risks and needs. A person expressing high levels of suicidal ideation, with intent to act on these and little ability to keep themselves safe will need a different more intensive care plan than someone who is self-harming as a coping strategy with no suicidal intent. It is however important to keep in mind research evidence about the relationship between self-harm and suicide. A history of self-harm is the biggest risk factor for suicide, and cutting has shown to carry greater risk of suicide than self-poisoning (Hawton et al. 2012) and that, over time, self-harm stops working as a coping strategy, so leading to hopelessness (Townsend et al. 2016a, b).

10.13 Care Plan, Safety Plan and Follow-Up

Following the assessment, an initial formulation is developed, from which a care plan can be agreed with the young person and their parents. After an episode of self-harm, the care plan will always include a safety plan as well as a plan to address underlying issues/needs, identifying which services are needed to do this. The young person will need to be referred to the most appropriate service for their needs, e.g. school nurses, third sector organisations (these may vary according to local provision and commissioning arrangements), or community CAMHS.

The nurse uses their knowledge of what the safety plan should consist of but also needs to use the above skills to collaborate with and engage the young person and parents in implementing the agreed plan. At times when young people, parents and professionals may have different views, and the plan is not agreed by all, this needs to be clearly documented.

A safety plan should include:

- Warning signs/triggers—thoughts, feelings, behaviours—the things that precede self-harm and contribute to the 'urge' to self-harm
- Safe storage of medicines and agreed plan re-sharps/safety in the home
- Alternative internal and external coping strategies: things that I can do—different thoughts and ways to cope with these triggers, dealing with the distress in a different way
- Family/friends who can support me when needed
- Professionals who can support me when needed
- Helplines/services I can contact
- List of positive things in my life
- Things I am looking forward to

On rare occasions, a young person may present with significantly high risk factors that result in the CAMH nurse deeming that it is not currently safe for the young person to return home or to be discharged from hospital. Depending on the reasons for this and whether they are predominately seen as being mental health or social care/safeguarding concerns, the young person is likely to remain in a general hospital bed until a multi-agency meeting is held the next day. This enables further assessment if needed and a more comprehensive multi-agency care plan to be agreed that may include the young person being discharged to alternative accommodation with extended family/friends or within the care system or admitted to a psychiatric adolescent unit. The CAMH nurse uses their communication and liaison skills in contributing to this process and decision-making by sharing their assessment findings and their understanding gained from the young person/family. These can often be difficult situations to navigate depending on the views of the young person and family but also sometimes because of differing opinions between professionals and agencies.

10.14   Communication Skills

How does all of this translate into practice, what do young people and families experience, what can student nurses and colleagues observe?

Listening skills; mental health nurses in CAMHS, like the Samaritans, operate on promoting the skill of active listening, usually opening up rather than closing down the conversation at the young person's pace, using skills of reflecting and clarifying. In other words listening to understand, Covey (1989) believes 'most people do not listen with the intent to understand; they listen with the intent to reply'.

Feeling listened to is consistently reported by young people as being critically important. Some organisations recognise this, with CAMH nurses routinely asking young people and parents for written feedback and then providing a response, reinforcing that they are listening via the iterative process (see examples of this, Figs. 10.2 and 10.3).

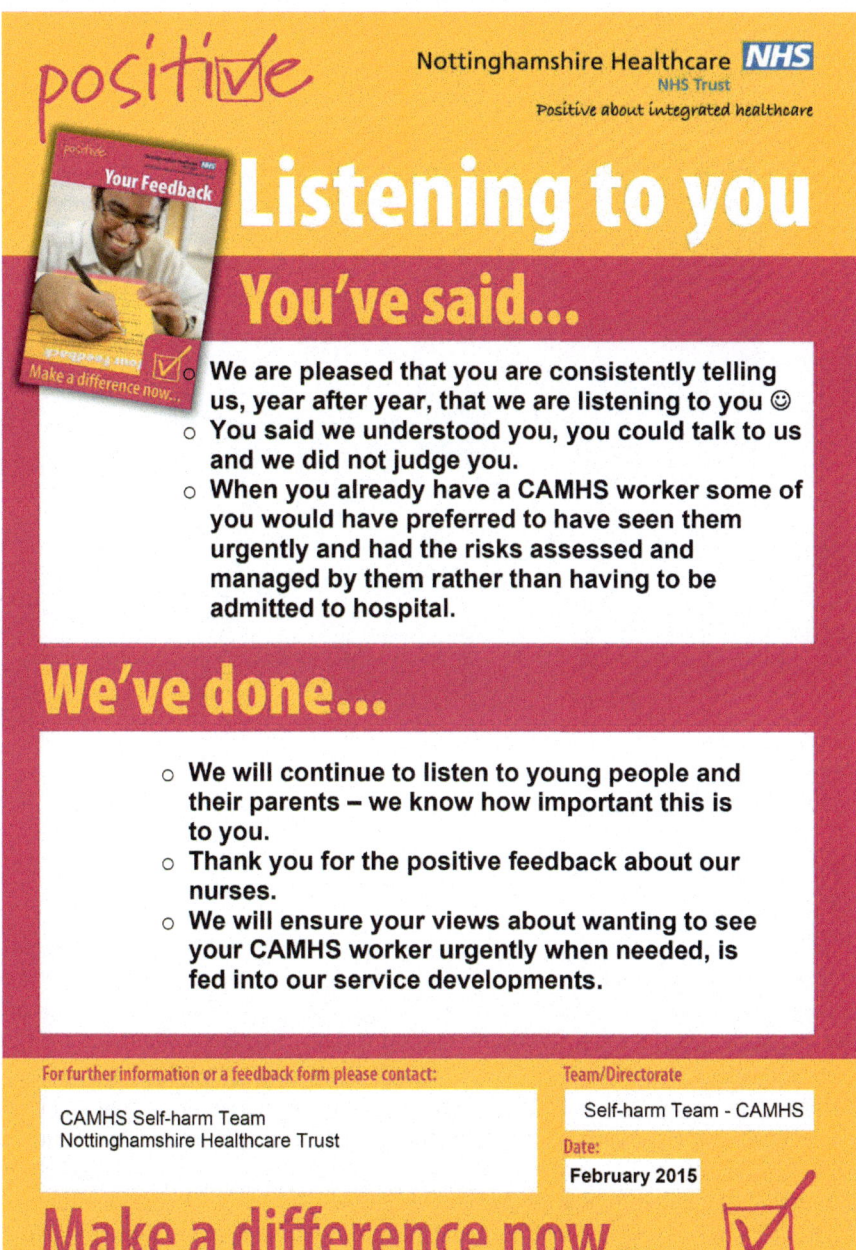

Fig. 10.2 Example of feedback system (used by kind permission of Notts Healthcare NHS FT)

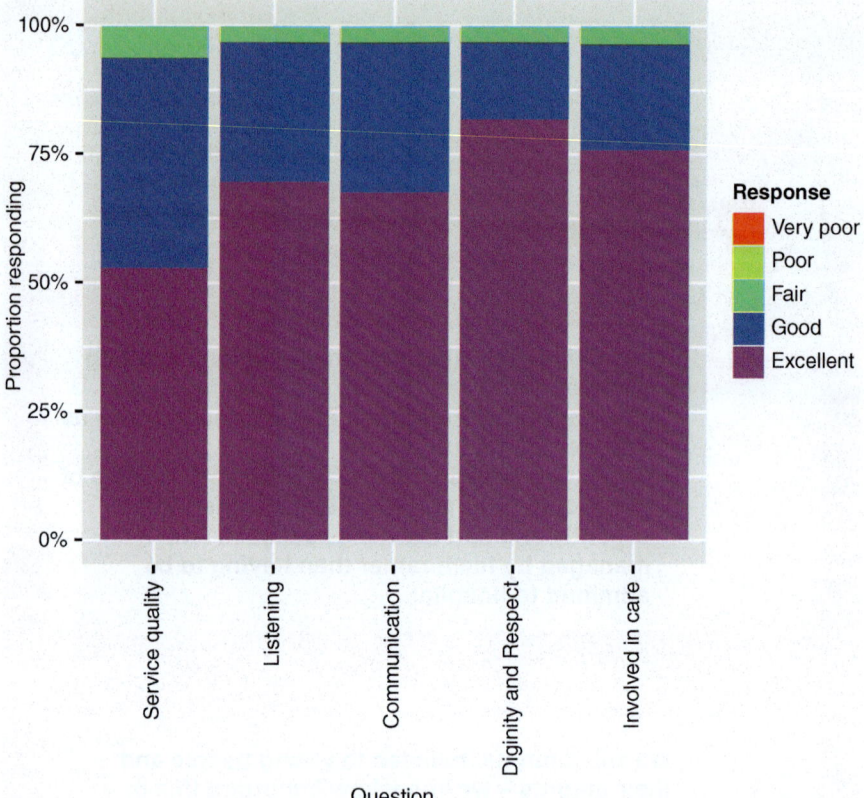

Fig. 10.3 Service user feedback on importance of interactional elements

Our non-verbal skills; eye contact, facial expression, gestures, body posture all give a thousand messages without a word being spoken. They indicate if we are interested, if we care, if we have time, young people are very astute at picking up any incongruences between what is being said verbally and non-verbally.

Many young people who self-harm have low self-esteem, so they may already doubt if they are 'worth' helping. This alongside possible low mood and negative thought patterns, e.g. ideas that they cannot be helped, or that things will not change/get better, can mean they tune into any clues including non-verbal communication strengthening their belief that people may be uninterested or indifferent about helping them. A recent study found that self-esteem, measured at baseline, predicted self-harm status at 6-month follow-up, and no other psychological variable predicted self-harm cessation (Townsend et al. 2016a, b).

All communications and interactions with young people require the CAMH nurse to be skilled in the area of questioning. Questions are the basis for gaining information which leads to an understanding of the self-harm, clarifying and deepening that understanding as well as forming the therapeutic relationship. The CAMH nurse needs skills in knowing when to use open and closed questions, for example they might ask an open question: 'Tell me how you were feeling at that time..', which would invite a detailed description, if the CAMH nurse judged that the young person seemed happy to talk and open up more. On the other hand, in exactly the same situation, but if the young person was struggling to stay in the room and was very upset, the CAMH nurse might ask a closed question, such as 'Did you feel sad?', believing this was all they could tolerate at that time.

As well as the episode of self-harm itself, and the underlying issues a young person may be struggling with, following the self-harm they often experience additional negative emotions such as guilt and shame. All this can add together to present a complex presentation that the CAMH nurse needs to understand.

Whilst clinical formulation is not part of mental health nurse training or the nursing process, it is commonly expected that CAMH nurses, alongside all members of the multi-disciplinary team, have the skills needed to use their theoretical knowledge to understand the clinical presentation from which to plan, implement and evaluate care.

The communication and interactions with the young person go beyond that of assessment. Young people tell us that when they have had a bad experience from services they are put off seeking further help; this can lead to them not attending further appointments; whilst on the contrary, a positive experience will encourage them to attend and seek further help in future if needed. It is important that the CAMH nurse uses their skills to portray a genuine position of acceptance and validation of the young person.

However short or long their relationship, their time in CAMHS, the CAMH nurse aims to help the young person by teaching them skills and techniques that can better equip them to understand and deal with possible future stresses. So the CAMH nurse is using the opportunity of the current presentation of self-harm to build resilience and future life skills.

10.15   Emotional Containment

Perhaps one of the most necessary and valued skills of CAMH nurses when working with young people who self-harm is that of emotional containment. Often when young people present with self-harm, they and/or their parents can be in a highly distressed state, hence the point of crisis and them feeling overwhelmed with their thoughts, emotions and their situation. This can occur immediately prior to the self-harm, and can still be present following self-harm, at the time of assessment and beyond. They may feel 'out of control' and unable to 'sit-with/be-with' their emotional state, though this has often reduced and become more bearable by the time of assessment.

When they bring that 'way of being' to the assessment, or later to the therapy/ intervention session, the reaction and response of the CAMH nurse is critical. The CAMH nurse needs to be able to relate to them in a way that provides a 'safe space', that conveys a sense of safety by calmly being with someone, listening, validating and responding, but not overreacting to their expression of distress. This, alongside clear boundaries, enables the young person to share their thoughts and feelings. As a prerequisite, the application of this skill requires the CAMH nurse to be competent in 'containing' their own emotions, in order to contain those of the young person and, where needed, their parents/family. The detail of achieving this goes beyond the remit of this chapter but includes the individual's ability to be self-aware, resilient and use their ability to reflect.

10.16   Parents/Carers

When a young person is in crisis, it is likely that the parent or parents feel they are in crisis too. Parents usually see their 'job' as 'protecting' their children, so when they discover they have self-harmed, or the self-harm has escalated to need hospital attendance, or the young person is expressing suicidal thoughts, this can feel very scary, a time of many mixed emotions including heightened anxiety. The CAMH nurse can signpost parents to literature, helping them understand self-harm and the common issues that parents of young people who self-harm experience, as well as interacting directly with them (McDougall et al. 2010).

Sometimes young people identify stresses within the family; contributing factors that they feel are having a negative impact on their emotional health and well-being. The CAMH nurse uses their communications skills, navigating and negotiating, to work on making changes in a way that keeps everyone engaged, promotes positive family relationships, and aids the young person's recovery. For example, it may be that a parent is struggling themselves; an important part of the assessment process would be identifying, liaising and signposting if a parent needed support, including with their own mental health.

In situations where there are safeguarding (child protection) concerns regarding the family, appropriate referrals would be made following organisational policy and procedures. A helpful model and framework for thinking about the different skills a CAMH nurse utilises in these situations is that of the three domains of action (Lang et al. 1990): (1) production—which would include following safeguarding procedures; (2) explanation - which would be the therapeutic space, and: (3) aesthetics - which is the way in which the nurse skilfully works across these domains.

Usually parents are young people's biggest resource and source of support. They advocate for the young person, addressing identified needs, help them to feel physically and emotionally safe and where possible bringing about changes needed in various aspects of the young person's life. Some services and localities will have parents support groups and other resources that parents can access. In these settings, parents are able to express their distress and share common experiences such as feeling they are 'walking on egg shells', being afraid to apply boundaries, and parent in their 'usual' way for fear of the young person self-harming when chastised. It is very common that parents blame themselves when their child self-harms; meeting other parents can help them to see this differently, as described here:

> *It didn't matter how often people told me it wasn't my fault, it felt like I had done something wrong. Then I met these other mums and dads, and guess what they were clever, and chatty, and funny, and seemed to be really good parents. I dared to think if it didn't occur to me that it was their fault then maybe it wasn't my fault either.* Julia—parent.

In this context, CAMH nurses apply their skills to the role of group facilitation. Providing the right environment and atmosphere, relaxed and welcoming— 'professionally friendly', being supportive and encouraging, giving everyone an opportunity to share and gain support.

10.17   Multi-Agency Working, Liaison and Building Professional Relationships

When assessing a young person on a general hospital paediatric ward, the skills of the CAMH nurse extends to supporting the paediatric team to safely manage the young person during their stay on the ward. The skills described above, gained from experience working on in-patient mental health settings, are valuable and transferable in terms of use of observations, supporting young people to feel safe and the de-escalation of difficult situations, behaviours and feelings.

Children's nurses, who have often received minimal training in mental health, need support from the CAMH nurses as they can find looking after young people on the ward who self-harm both scary and anxiety provoking. As a means of caring for these young people, they need to assess and ensure their safety; a tool has recently been developed to help identify immediate risk of self-harm and suicidality in young people presenting to acute paediatric care (Manning et al. 2018).

An important part of keeping a young person safe, and helping them 'recover', is ensuring that the right professionals are aware and informed about what they need to know in a timely manner, and that relevant information is shared between services. This involves communicating relevant information via letter or referral form, and/or via telephone conversation. This may include following policy such as a referral to social care where there are child protection or safeguarding concerns, or about good practice, e.g. requesting a GP contributes to a safety plan with safe prescribing of a medication, which may mean a different choice of medication and/or prescribing smaller quantities. It may also refer to the additional support that schools can offer with, for example, get out of lesson passes, allocated mentors and time in school support centre.

Building good relationships with other professionals helps to ensure multiagency care plans are agreed and implemented. Understanding the roles and constraints of other organisations enables honest dialogue and promotes the use of informal consultation with multi-agencies working together to support the young person.

10.18   Documentation and IT Skills

When thinking about the skills of the CAMH nurse, this does not stop at the face to face skills utilised whilst in the direct care setting. There is a huge administration function attached to role, requiring skills previously not needed. This includes IT skills for electronic note keeping, routine use of standardised outcomes measures, and the use of various apps and programmes providing digital information to young people and families.

10.19   Learning the Skills Named in This Chapter

We learn and develop our skills through practice; it can help to observe others and possibly find a mentor or role model, someone whose skills we admire and want to achieve. It also helps to reflect on our own experiences, times when for example we have felt listened to, what was it that the person did that made us feel heard? By doing this, we make connections and see the importance of the skill we are practising and trying to accomplish. It may be that we are more skilled in certain circumstances but less skilled in others, e.g. we find it easier to actively listen when the person is highly distressed talking about loss following bereavement, and more difficult when they are talking about self-harm. Whilst it may be uncomfortable and take us out of our comfort zone, it is in these areas that we need more practice to build our skills.

10.20   Feedback

So how do you know if you are using the above skills effectively and areas where you could improve? We may already be self-aware and know some areas where we need to build our skills. Using self-reflexivity, reflecting both 'in' and 'on' action (Schön 1983) are important skills not only for clinical assessment and therapeutic work but also for professional development and developing our skills.

An example of reflecting 'in action' would be noticing in the clinical session that a young person seems to have become less communicative, is starting to give one word answers and take longer to respond than usual. Feeding this back to the young person at the time, from a non-judgemental position of curiosity, opened up a conversation about the young person feeling exhausted having had very little sleep the night before. This led to further information about why the young person had not slept and their current worries.

An example of reflecting 'on action' would be discussing the above session in clinical supervision and reporting how the young person's responses had changed. Reflecting on why this may be, forming ideas and hypothesis that can then be either kept in mind or shared with the young person at the next session.

Forums such as clinical supervision also give a supportive space, for example to talk about an occasion when you have felt less compassionate towards a young person than you would usually, the possible reasons and influences for this.

Mentorship and getting feedback from colleagues either formally through appraisal/360 feedback, or informally, and recording and reviewing our sessions also provide opportunities to review and reflect on our practice and skills. For example, when reviewing our practice we/others may notice that we interrupt or offer suggested solutions more than we thought. Over time, it may also provide an opportunity for evidencing change, improvements and developments in our skills.

Obtaining regular feedback both verbal and written from young people and parents is another source of valuable information—see example on enclosed poster Fig. 10.2.

It might be after the crisis has passed and the young person and family are in a happier place that they are more able to reflect on their experience. For most CAMH nurses positive feedback from young people and families is the best part about their job, the reason they do their job, for example having them say:

> You saved my life/our family; I don't know what we would have done without you

It is so often what seems like the smallest of considerations that make the biggest differences.

10.21   Summary

In summary, CAMH nurses bring skills of care and compassion, develop a therapeutic relationship by listening and being non-judgemental, and are skilled in identifying and managing mental health problems. They get 'alongside' young people to work in collaboration with them and their families in helping them understand and manage or move on from self-harm.

Thanks to all the young people and parents, including those that have contributed to this chapter, who have helped me develop my skills through the therapeutic relationships created with them and the valuable feedback given by them.

References

Baldwin L (2008) The discourse of professional identity in child and adolescent mental health services. PhD thesis, University of Nottingham. Access from the University of Nottingham repository http://eprints.nottingham.ac.uk/10504/1/LBaldwinThesis2008.pdf

Callaghan P, Gamble C (eds) (2015) Oxford handbook of mental health nursing, 2nd edn. Oxford University Press, Oxford

Callaghan P, Playle J, Cooper L (eds) (2009) Mental health nursing skills. Oxford University Press, Oxford

Covey SR (1989) The 7 habits of highly effective people: powerful lessons in personal change. Free Press, New York

DH (2012) Compassion in practice: nursing, midwifery and care staff our vision and strategy December. Published to www.commissioningboard.nhs.uk in electronic format only

Fruggeri L (2012) Different levels of psychotherapeutic competence. J Fam Ther 34(1):91–105

Gray AJ (2002) Stigma in psychiatry. J R Soc Med 95(2):72–76

Hawton K, Bergen H, Kapur N, Cooper J, Steeg S, Ness J, Waters K (2012) Repetition of self-harm and suicide following self-harm in children and adolescents: findings from the multicentre study of self-harm in England. J Child Psychol Psychiatry 53:1212–1219

Horvath AO (2001) The alliance. Psychother Theory Res Pract Train 38(4):365–372

Kapur N (2017). https://www.youtube.com/watch?v=fpmSqTQNeHc. Accessed 26 Apr 2019

Lang WP, Little M, Cronen V (1990) The systemic professional: domains of action and the question of neutrality. Human Syst J Syst Consult Manag 1:39–56

Manning JC, Walker GM, Carter T, Aubeeluck A, Witchell M, Coad J (2018) Children & Young People Mental Health Safety Assessment Tool (CYPMH SAT) study: protocol for the development and psychometric evaluation of an assessment tool to identify immediate risk of self-harm and suicide in children and young people (10–19 years) in acute paediatric hospital settings. BMJ Open 8:e020964. https://doi.org/10.1136/bmjopen-2017-02096

McDougall T, Armstrong M, Trainor G (2010) Helping children and young people who self-harm: an introduction to self-harming and suicidal behaviours for health professionals. Routledge, London

National Collaborating Centre for Mental Health (NCCMH) (2018) Self-harm and suicide prevention competence framework: children and young people. Health Education England, London

National Collaborating Centre of Mental Health (NCCMH) (2016) Achieving better access to 24/7 urgent and emergency mental health care. Part 4: implementing the evidence-based treatment pathway for Mental Health Services for Children and Young People. NHS England, London

National Institute for Health and Clinical Excellence (NICE) (2004) Self-harm: the short-term physical and psychological management and secondary prevention of self-harm in primary and secondary care (NICE Clinical Guidance 16). NICE, London

Nursing and Midwifery Council (NMC) (2018) The code: professional standards of practice and behaviour for nurses, midwives and nursing associates. NMC, London

Peplau HE (1952) Interpersonal relations in nursing. G P Putnam, New York

Rogers C (1951) Client-centred therapy: its current practice, implications and theory. Constable, London

Schön D (1983) The reflective practitioner: how professionals think in action. Temple Smith, London

Townsend E, Wadman R, Sayal K, Armstrong M, Harroe C, Majumder P (2016a) Uncovering key patterns in self-harm in adolescents: sequence analysis using the Card Sort Task for Self-harm (CaTS). J Affect Disord 206:161–168

Townsend E, Wadman R, Berry A, Sawyer C, Sayal K, Armstrong M, Harroe C, Majumder P, Vostanis P Clarke D (2016b) The 'listen-up!' project: understanding and helping looked-after young people who self-harm. Final report. Department of Health Policy Research Programme Project 023/0164

Chapter 11
Helping Children and Young People Understand Issues of Consent to Treatment

Ann Marie Cox

11.1 Consent Overview

Consent is a process that should be legally ensured in every aspect of CAMHS that relates to a child or young person (CYP) or their family; it is a continual process and is not a one-off event. This can be a difficult process to negotiate within the family orientated philosophy of CAMHS (CAMHS 2008). In any event, consent should not be assumed. The option of withdrawing or changing the parameters of consent should be a frequent conversation the nurse should have with the person who is giving consent. Consent should be gained by the nurse, at each and every contact with or about a CYP or family member (Department of Health (DH) 2009), in or outside of the CAMH service. The importance of involving CYP in their own care has become a priority in recent years throughout CAMHS (CAMHS 2008; DH 2003). We must ensure consent is gained from the CYP, or family member to undertake any intervention in CAMHS and to share the necessary information with the external professionals or services. When CAMHS sends information out about a CYP's mental health, the nurse should be asking who should the letters be addressed to. It should not be automatic that letters are only sent to the parents. The recording and documentation of consent is also a necessity that nurses should do with great diligence (Cox et al. 2017). There are some rare exceptions when consent is not needed to share information. These are when you are processing information in order to fulfil a legal obligation, such as safeguarding children or reporting a crime or protecting the general public, for which you are covered for by article 6.1.C under the GDPR (The European Parliament and the Council of the European Union 2016).

Consent is defined as an agreement or approval to do something or giving the permission or allowing for something to happen. We are bound by the English law (Department of Health (DH) 2009); the Data Protection Act, (U. K. Government

A. M. Cox (✉)
North Staffordshire Combined NHS Trust, North Staffordshire, UK

© Springer Nature Switzerland AG 2020
L. Baldwin (ed.), *Nursing Skills for Children and Young People's Mental Health*,
https://doi.org/10.1007/978-3-030-18679-1_11

2018) and the associated General Data Protection Regulations (The European Parliament and the council of the European Union 2016) to ensure that we gain consent for any intervention we use with a CYP or family member and what we do with the information we elicit through the process.

Informed consent is based upon three principles, these being

- To understanding treatment options and the associated risk and benefits
- That it is made voluntarily and in the absence of any pressure or coercion
- That there is a presence of capacity (Tan et al. 2007; Wellesley and Jenkins 2009)

Many theorists posit the need for nurses to be skilled in the assessment and process of seeking consent (Alderson 2007; Boyden 2005; Boylan and Braye 2006; Donnelly 2010; Tan and Fegert 2004; Tan et al. 2007). However, the literature to evidence what specific training nurses need to undertake and what skills should be taught is extremely limited (Cox et al. 2016). There has been some recent work by the Anna Freud National Centre for Children and Families, around shared decision-making with young people; however, this does not explicitly cover whether a CYP is able to consent for themselves but describes to the process of making the decision between clinician, CYP and family member, where necessary, rather than considering whether the CYP has the ability to consent (Abrines-Jaume et al. 2016; CAMHS Evidenced based Practice Unit (EBPU) 2014).

The CAMH service should have consent forms that specifically request consent for sharing information about CYPs and their families. This will usually include the CYP's school, other professionals already involved with the CYP and a caveat that incorporates other necessary professionals. The consent for the sharing of information needs to be sought at the very first contact with the CYP, so you are clear about what services and professionals you have been given permission to speak with. It is helpful to remember that this information solely relates to the CYP being supported by CAMHS and not any other members of the family; therefore, if you wish to discuss other members of the family, then you must gain separate consent for these; again, this may not be required in specific safeguarding situations. When the sharing of information is discussed, there should also be an explicit discussion about how you as a professional will be using the information you elicit through contact with the CYP, and explain how it will be used and discussed including with members of the team and in supervision. It is important that CYP and families know what is happening with their information and how it will be used as directed by the General Data Protection Regulations (GDPR) and they are in agreement with the use of the information (The European Parliament and the Council of the European Union 2016; U.K. Government 2018).

This chapter will detail the current landscape regarding consent and offer an understanding of contemporary CYP and parental rights. There will be an overview of case law and legal implications that impact on consent and decision-making. Finally, a consideration of child development factors will be considered; however, a more in-depth review of child development is available in Chap. 3. The chapter will then offer some skills that can be used in gaining consent and how to record it ensuring it is valid.

Learning Point Summary
- Every contact with or about a CYP or family member needs to have valid consent.
- Ensure that consent is gained for sharing and discussing information at all levels of CAMHS care.
- There may be times when consent is not needed when you are fulfilling a legal obligation, such as reporting a child safeguarding concern or protecting the public from harm.
- The recording and documenting of consent is as important as gaining it.
- CYP and families can withdraw consent at any time.

11.2   Case Law and Consent

There are a number of case law outcomes that can be helpful to consider in the context of consent and in how it has developed over time. Bolam v Friern Hospital Management Committee (1957) was an influential outcome that has provided a foundation for all recent case law outcomes to be compared against. Bolam was a psychiatric patient who was undergoing Electro Convulsive Therapy (ECT). However, the doctor that gave the ECT did not use a muscle relaxant and Bolam received a broken pelvis amongst other injuries. A test was developed to consider whether the doctor who gave the ECT was negligent in his duties. As the consensus in the medical profession at that time was not in favour of using muscle relaxants; and that the majority of the doctor's peers would not have used a muscle relaxant; the outcome of the case deemed that the doctor had done what 'any reasonable competent practitioner would do'. It was found that the doctor was not negligent (Ibid). There have been criticisms of the Bolam conclusion, with one criticism being that the legal system relinquished power to the medical profession (MaClean 2002). Further case law subsequent to the Bolam case has been influential within the consent context, these being Sidaway v Board of Governors of the Bethlem Royal Hospital 1985, Simms v Simms 2003, R v Bournewood Community and Mental Health NHS Trust (1997), Bolitho v City and Hackney Health Authority (1997) and Montgomery vs. NHS Lanarkshire (Royal College of Gynaecologists 2016); the outcomes of these cases have observed a swing of the power move back to the courts in determining what is reasonable practice. This is an ever-changing landscape that impacts on safeguards for the nurse around gaining consent, so it is important to keep abreast of current case law outcomes.

11.3   Child Rights

Child rights have been relatively slow to develop in the UK in comparison to other European countries (Humanium 2010; Jones and Welch 2010). More recently over the past decade, there has been a significant emphasis in hearing the child's voice and ensuring their participation (Jones and Welch 2010) throughout services that CYPs are in contact with. Participation strategies are now well recognised as necessary throughout all health, social care and educational domains (Chitsabesan 2018; National Children's Bureau 2019). CYP's Improving Access to Psychological Therapies (CYP-IAPT) which commenced in 2011 is the current strategy that all CAMHS services in England have to ensure they are compliant with by 2020. CYP-IAPT has participation as one of its five main principals and embeds participation central to all levels of service delivery (NHS England (NHSE) 2018). Other significant rights are obliged through the United Nations Convention on the Rights of the Child (UNCRC) (1989), the Children Act (1989 & 2004) and the Human Rights Act (1998). What is clear through these mandates is that CYP's views have to be heard and clinicians have to ensure that they facilitate views being heard. This may mean the clinician has to be creative to ensure that the CYP can communicate their views fully. As it is a legal obligation to involve children in their own care, by not doing so, the nurse will be committing a criminal offence.

In supporting CYP to participate in session and share their views, the use of pictures, books and other communication resources can be helpful. Using such resources to help the CYP understand their options and consent to what they want to happen, or at the very least be part of the decision-making process is important in ensuring that they have participated in their fullest capacity; the 'mefirst' website (http://www.mefirst.org.uk/) (Great Ormond Street Hospital for Children NHS Foundation Trust and The Common Room 2019) has resources to help such communication. There are some further resources towards the end of this chapter. One aspect that has been evidenced to help CYPs become more involved in decision-making and consent processes is the child's previous experience. The more experience the CYP has in this area of practice, the more confident they will be in it. With the nurse taking care and time in the first instance of CYPs being involved in consent and decision-making processes, this will significantly help the CYP develop confidence and will significantly improve their involvement in subsequent events. It is essential that enough time is offered in involving CYPs in a process that is meaningful and supportive, laying a foundation for further involvement.

Paul et al. (2000) found in their research that a very high proportion of CYP who attended their healthcare appointments had not actually consented to attend and were in attendance through parental coercion. It is important to clarify if CYP understands why they are coming to CAMHS and ensure that they consent, if able to do so, in being there. In England, there is not a specific age that has been set with regards when a child may be able to be competent to consent (Information Commissioners Office 2018). Many theorists have argued that all assessments of competency for capacity should be undertaken in consideration of the stage of development of the child and not chronological age, with the phrase 'stage not age' being a helpful reminder (Didcock 2007; Donnelly 2010; Larcher and Hutchinson 2009; Parekh 2006; Tan and Fegert 2004). The onus therefore lies upon the nurse to demonstrate whether a child is competent and therefore is able to make an informed decision. Any child of any age can consent to a decision if they can demonstrate having competence and capacity. The nurse will need to use negotiating skills and support the CYP in being involved in decision-making and consent processes; at times the nurse may need to see the CYP individually to empower and give the greatest opportunity to be involved. At times the family orientated approach in CAMHS can be disempowering for CYPs to be as fully involved in decision-making and consent processes as possible, this can be due to expectations and agendas of other persons attending the appointment (Tan et al. 2007); however, ensuring all familial views are heard is mutually important.

Young people aged 16 years and over start from a position of being deemed to have capacity (Mental Capacity Act (MCA) 2005) whilst children under the aged of 16 are deemed not to. This is because the MCA (2005) refers to all people aged 16 years and over. For a young person 16 years and older, it is the nurse's responsibility to determine whether the young person lacks capacity (due to the young person deemed to have capacity in the eyes of the law). In the nurse's role of gaining consent of a child under the age of 16, the nurse has to determine whether the CYP demonstrates capacity and competence to do so. If a CYP is deemed not to have capacity or competence, then consent is not informed and will not be valid in this instance. The CYP's capacity and competence may change in the future, so it will be important to ensure this is revisited to establish whether the CYP can consent at a future date. It is also important to remember that consent and capacity are decision and time specific, therefore at another time or for another decision, the CYP may have capacity and competence (MCA 2005; DH 2009). In the event of the CYP not being able to consent, it will be extremely important that the CYP continues to be involved in the decision-making process and shares their views as much as possible. In these situations, informed consent should be gained from a parent or caregiver that has Parental Responsibility (PR) (Information Commissioners Office 2018). However, too much alignment with parental views can leave CYPs feeling demoralised (Donnelly 2010) and can significantly hinder CYP's involvement and participation (Boylan and Braye 2006). A significant difference that nurses need to be aware of regarding consent is that CYPs under the age of 16 years are not able to refuse treatment (DH 2009). This area of practice raises real concerns in the child rights debate, as it raises the question whether CYPs under the age of 16 years do hold full rights if they can only consent to treatment and not refuse it (Al-Samsam 2008; Parekh 2006). This offers opportunity for the nurse to be creative when supporting CYPs under 16 years, in that offering several options of treatment or avenues of support will help reduce the possibility of the CYPs wanting to refuse treatment, giving them more self-agency and autonomy in their care. However, there is an importance on ensuring involvement in decision-making and consent processes is not burdensome on the CYP and causes more stress than empowerment (Alderson and Montgomery 1996; Cantwell and Scott 1995; Billick et al. 1998).

There are two main frameworks that support CYP; these are the MCA (2005) for those children aged 16 years and over and the Gillick competency framework (Gillick v Norfolk and Wisbech Health Authority 1985) for those under 16 years. We will consider these two legal frameworks in more depth.

11.4   The Mental Capacity Act

The MCA (2005) is an act of law that discusses all aspects of capacity and competence relating to those 'persons who are unable make a decision because of an impairment of, or disturbance in the functioning of, the mind or brain' (Part 1, section 2 (1), MCA 2005). This definition includes any physical and psychological reasons for any impairment, whether it is a temporary or permanent loss of capacity. The exclusions from the MCA are murder, suicide and supported suicide (Part 3, section 62, MCA 2005).

The MCA (2005) defines what a person needs to be able in order to be deemed competent and have capacity to make a decision. These four main criterions are:

    (a) to understand the information relevant to the decision
    (b) to retain that information
    (c) to use or weigh that information as part of the process of making the decision
    or
    (d) to communicate his decision (whether by talking, using sign language or any other means. (Part, section 3 (1), MCA 2005)

The use of this four-point standard can be a helpful format when documenting and recording the conversation that has taken place to ascertain whether a CYP has or lacks capacity. It assists in demonstrating that each criterion has been explicitly discussed and will demonstrate how the evidence from the discussion informs the overall judgement on whether a person has capacity has been reached.

11.5   Gillick Competency Framework

The Gillick competency framework (Gillick v Norfolk and Wisbech Health Authority 1985) is based on an outcome of a court case. Victoria Gillick took Norwich and Wisbech Health authority to court after a circular from the Department of Health and Social security (DHSS) advised that CYP under the age of 16 could have a discussion about contraception with a General Practitioner (GP) without the need for parental consent. The discussion about contraception would be at the GP's discretion if it was deemed that the test for capacity was met. Mrs Gillick disagreed with this and felt children should not be able to consent to contraception and that parents should have the overriding consent about what happens with their children aged under 16 years. In the court hearing, Lord Scarman stated that

> As a matter of law, the parental right to determine whether or not their minor child below the age of sixteen will have medical treatment terminates if and when the child achieves sufficient understanding and intelligence to understand fully what is proposed (Gillick v Norfolk and Wisbech Health Authority 1985).

The following outcome was upheld from the Gillick hearing,

> A girl under the age of 16 had the legal capacity to consent to medical examination and treatment, including contraceptive treatment, if she had sufficient maturity and intelligence

to understand the nature and implications of the treatment. The rights of parents to determine such matters ended when a child achieved sufficient intelligence and understanding to
make her own decision (Gillick v Norwich and Wisbech Health Authority 1985).

These criterions are only slightly different from the MCA (2005) criterion, with the inclusion of intelligence. Arguably, this could be a factor in any age of patient, including adults. Ensuring that the 'stage not age' phrase is considered in all situations will be a good foundation for ensuring assessments of capacity and competence are as objective as possible. Personally held values, assumptions and prejudices of the capacity or competence assessor need to be held in the forefront of the mind to aid the objectivity (Alderson 2007; James and Prout 1997). An example of this is that you may hold the assumption that all parents have capacity, when some might not; or you may think that because a CYP doesn't speak, they won't have competence or capacity; the nurse may need to find creative ways of working with the CYP to assess competence or capacity that is non-verbal. This may be through writing, drawing, developing resources such as story boards, to help involve them and assess their competence and capacity.

The Gillick case also developed the Fraser Guidelines. Fraser guidelines and the Gillick competency framework frequently get confused. The two are not interchangeable, so it is important that you use the correct framework when assessing competence. In the Gillick case, Lord Fraser did offer guidance about decision-making and competence for under 16-year-olds, but this was specifically related to contraception. Gillick is used more widely to assess competence in all instances (Wheeler 2006).

Whilst the MCA (2005) criterions are helpful as a foundation for assessing capacity, Griffith (2016, p. 245) offers the following criterion to support the assessment for legal competence. Griffith suggests that a child will only be considered legally competent once the following have been demonstrated:

- A level of maturity
- That the child is able to recognise, understand and manage external pressures from family, peers, society and pre-judgements with regard the decision being made
- A level of intelligence
- That the child can demonstrate a good understanding of the entirety of the decision, be able to balance the benefits and costs both in the short and long term and all in consideration the social, home and educational aspects of their lives.
- Griffith (2016, p. 245)

Gaining consent can be difficult in some circumstances, especially where there are conflicting agendas and when CYPs are deemed to have capacity and consent. As detailed in the outcome of the Gillick case (Gillick v Norfolk and Wisbech Health Authority 1985), 'the rights of parents to determine such matters ended when a child achieved sufficient intelligence and understanding to make her own decision'. As a nurse working in CAMHS, you have to remember the decisions made in CAMHS will affect the CYP at home. It is important that negotiating skills are used to help keep calmness and conflict to a minimum. It is these skills that are most important in these situations; in not achieving this, there is a possibility the CYP could go home to a very difficult and tense environment, subsequently impacting on the CYP's mental health.

Learning Point Summary
- All children should be heard. Even if they cannot give informed consent, their views should be included as much as possible.
- Potentially any child could consent, age should not determine whether a child can consent, it should be determined on 'stage not age'
- For 16 years and over, use the Mental Capacity Act (2005).
- For under 16s, use the Gillick competency framework.
- Under 16s cannot refuse treatment (Gillick v Norfolk and Wisbech Health Authority 1985); if a child does refuse, then this could be overridden by a person with PR.
- Negotiation skills are fundamental in supporting CYP to consent.
- Be creative in helping CYP share their views.
- Be aware of your own personally held values, assumptions and prejudices and how these may influence this area of practice.

11.6   Parental Rights (PR)

It is important that parents are involved as part of the decision-making process (Tan et al. 2007). Those with PR have continued responsibility for their children until 18 years of age under the Children Act (1989 & 2004). This conflict between the different legal mandates, for example, the Children Act (1989 & 2004) and Gillick competency framework (Gillick v Norfolk and Wisbech Health Authority 1985) can be difficult to negotiate. By nurses using their negotiating skills in balancing the views of CYP and their families, this can provide the most satisfactory of outcomes. In remembering that as the CYP will remain within the family dynamics, in reaching a consensus and having commitment to both CYP and the person with parental consent, it will improve collaborative participation and reduce the risk of further disagreements and confrontation at home (Cox et al. 2016; Boylan and Braye 2006).

In the event of a CYP not being able to give informed consent, you will have to seek consent from a parent or a caregiver with PR, it is important that you ensure that they have the correct permission to do so, and that they have capacity to consent themselves. All mothers are automatically given PR status. Most fathers if married to the mother or are detailed on the birth certificate also will have PR. There can be more than two people that hold PR for a child, so it is important to ascertain who these are (UK Government 2018).

Learning Point Summary
- Be clear about who has PR.
- There can be more than two people with PR for a child or young person.

- Those who have PR should be involved in consent processes.
- Nurses have a role in the negotiation of the consent and decision-making process in order to achieve a collaborative outcome

11.7   Children and Young People Accessing CAMHS Without Parental Consent or Knowledge

CYP accessing CAMHS without parental knowledge and consent can be an area of contention. Based on the information detailed in this chapter, legally, CYP can access CAMHS without parental consent. There are many valid reasons as to why a CYP may want to do this; this may relate to personal privacy; difficulties within the family dynamics that are impacting on the CYP's mental health; there may be abuse within the family home that the CYP is dealing with; the CYP may feel safer to talk to professionals without parents or caregivers being there. It is important that access to CAMHS is available for CYPs in the absence of parents or caregivers. That being said, understanding the CYP's rationale for not including parents or caregivers and understanding the associated risks is an important as part of the initial assessment. By parents not having knowledge about their child's involvement in CAMHS, could incur more risks and acrimony within the family, especially if the family are accidently made aware. You should document the risks about not sharing information with parents and caregivers (Care Quality Commission 2017). It is for the nurse to balance these risks and continue to support the CYP's engagement in CAMHS as much as possible. When these situations occur, developing a safety plan with the CYP is helpful; clearly explaining the bounds of confidentiality and potentially identifying an adult, not necessarily an adult with PR, that the CYP would allow for them to know that they are attending CAMHS are useful interventions to undertake. In any contact with CYP, you should always gain consent for information sharing, this may relate to letters being sent from CAMHS containing the CYP's mental health information and who these should be addressed to. This is particularly pertinent when CYPs are attending CAMHS without parents' consent, you do not want a letter going to the parents by default, when the parents are not involved. You should always revisit involving parents and caregivers and those with PR frequently throughout the CYP's episode of care. Clearly wherever there are safeguarding concerns, these need to be reported in line with legal processes in any event (The European Parliament and the Council of the European Union 2016).

Learning Point Summary
- CYP can access CAMHS without parental consent or knowledge.
- Support the CYP in helping you understand why they feel parents cannot be involved.
- Develop a safety plan with the CYP so everyone is clear how they are going to keep safe.
- Identify another adult that the CYP is happy for you to speak to.

- Identify how information should be sent to the CYP, they may want it sent to school or a different address
- Revisit involving parents or those with PR frequently.
- Report safeguarding concerns as necessary.

11.8　Recording and Documenting of Consent

The recording and documenting of consent is extremely important. Not only is it a legal obligation but it also should detail how you have demonstrated that a CYP has capacity to consent or not (Cox et al. 2017; DH 2009; MCA 2005). Cox et al. (2017) developed a checklist from the best available guidance and legal evidence. Figure 11.1 offers an adapted version of the checklist which includes the detail required to fully document consent. It is important to bear all of the checklist points in mind when documenting consent. As consent is an ongoing process, the nurse will not have to document all of the points on the checklist every time when revisiting consent for the *same* intervention. The nurse can refer back to the original consent gained for the intervention and advise that all points have been discussed and consent and capacity remain the same. The nurse must document that the responses gained for the original consent still stand and document any changes to the original responses.

Learning Point Summary
- The nurse should always ensure the checklist is fully completed in the first conversation about consent for each specific intervention.
- If it is not recorded, it will not be deemed as completed in a court of law.
- Whilst the first recording of consent is more detailed, this will support the nurse in future conversations about consent as this can be referred to and only changes to the consent need to be documented in detail; the rest can be agreed as remaining unchanged.
- Ensure that you revisit consent regularly and who has capacity and competence and document any relevant changes, including withdrawals of consent.

11.9　Nursing and Midwifery Council (NMC) Code of Conduct and Consent

The current conduct which was published by the NMC (2015) and can be found at this web address (https://www.nmc.org.uk/standards/code/read-the-code-online/) has four main sections within it 'prioritise people, practise effectively, preserve safety and promote professionalism and trust'. All four sections have aspects within them that would impact on an aspect of gaining, recording or documenting consent. It is helpful for the nurse to be mindful that they are not only upholding legal rights when involving CYPs in decision-making and consent processes, they are also upholding their professional rights too.

1)	Which nurse has discussed consent?
2)	What intervention is consent being sought for (be specific)?
3)	Which person is giving consent? (CYP, Person with PR?)
4)	Who else was present in the appointment?
5)	Is the nurse who discussed consent, going to provide the intervention?
6)	If it is another clinician that will provide the intervention, does the nurse who is gaining consent have sufficient knowledge about the intervention to explain the detail for consent purposes?
7)	Detail how consent was discussed and what resources were used? Did there need to be an interpreter for example, was this verbal or non-verbal, what worksheets or visual component were used to help the CYP be involved in consenting or decision making?
8)	How has capacity been assessed?
9)	Have they shown that the child can: (a) Understand the information that is given to them is relevant to the decision? (b) Retain information long enough to make a decision? (c) Use or weigh up the information as part of the decision-making process? (d) Communicate their decision?
10)	Did the discussion include (a) What sort of things will be involved in the treatment? (b) What benefits would the child hope to receive? (c) How good are the chances of getting such benefits? (d) What are the alternatives? (e) What are the risks, if any? (f) If there are any risks, are they minor or serious? (g) What may happen if the intervention is refused?
11)	Was there opportunity to discuss the above more than once?
12)	Is there anything getting in the way of informed consent? Eg: anxiety, pain, family members with different agendas
13)	Has the consent been given voluntarily and without coercion?
14)	Has there been a discussion about being able to withdraw consent?
15)	If the CYP is unable to give consent, how have they been participating in the decision-making process?
16)	Who decided best interests for the child? What was taken into consideration for best interests? (This should be a wide range of people who know the CYP, teachers, GP, friends etc. If applicable)
17)	Is the record keeping only captured once?
18)	Has the documentation of consent and capacity demonstrated that the decision is based on all available evidence?
19)	Is the consent form completed on the electronic patient record system (or specific form if not electronic)?
20)	Has the consent been discussed on more than one occasion?

Fig. 11.1 The recording and documenting of consent checklist (Adapted from Cox et al. 2017)

11.10   Resources

This last section will offer a range of resources to help with facilitating consent for CYPs. These are for the nurse to use to support the CYP and their families in understanding the information and establishing capacity and competence.

11.11   Circles of Compromise

Managing disagreements or competing agendas is one of the most commonplace difficulties seen in CAMHS when deciding on treatment options for CYPs. One simple way to negotiate an outcome is to use the following 'circles of compromise' tool in Fig. 11.2.

The circles of compromise are a helpful tool that can be used with CYPs and their parent, caregiver or family to come to a compromise about treatment options. This tool does not negate the position of competence or capacity but is helpful to use if there is a concern that the CYP will be at an increased risk of distress in returning home due to the competing agendas or differences of opinion. As previously highlighted, it is important to ensure that the CYP is not further distressed due to the decisions agreed within CAMHS. On using the circles of compromise, the nurse can draw these circles on a big sheet of paper or a white board to use to support the intervention. By making the drawing visible to everyone, this helps with a collaborative approach to the intervention. Start off by adding in the CYP's views on treatment in circle one and the parental and caregiver's views in circle two; some example have been added in Fig. 11.2 to offer some ideas. Then you use circle three to draw up a compromise and an agreement between both competing views. How might you negotiate the compromise in circle three in this situation detailed in Fig. 11.2?

An example of a compromise in this instance that could be detailed in circle three:

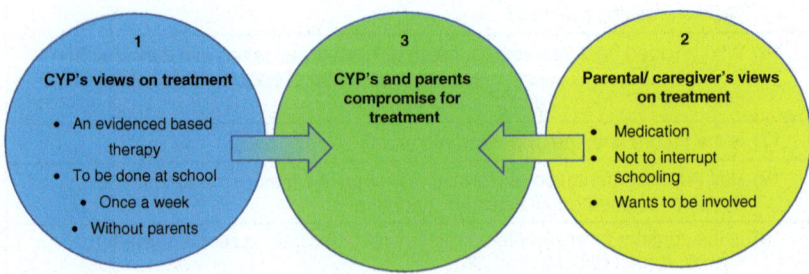

Fig. 11.2 The circles of compromise

- *An evidenced based therapy will be offered to begin with* This would be evidence-based therapy detailed in the National Institute of Health and Care Excellence (NICE) guidance (NICE 2019). Education about treatments is extremely helpful for both CYPs and the parents and caregivers in order for them to make informed choices; this would include evidence-based therapies and pharmacological treatments. Many CYPs and caregivers do not fully understand the concepts and structures of evidence-based therapies, or understand the side effects or pharmacokinetics of medication. For example, when being prescribed some mainstream anti-depressants such as Selective Serotonin Reuptake Inhibitors (SSRIs) with examples such as fluoxetine and sertraline, there is not much knowledge around the potential side effects of suicidal ideation and that they can take up to 12 weeks to have full impact. Many believe that all medication work with immediate effect (NHS 2019).
- *It will take place in school, but on alternative lessons.* To understand the CYP's and parent/caregivers' perspective in why they do or do not want it to take place in school is an important understanding for the nurse. In this instance, the CYP struggled with transport and found it difficult to get to CAMHS premises and wanted to support themselves under their own volition; parents did not want the CYP to miss any lessons due to upcoming exams and concerns about the CYP missing too much of the same lesson. Therefore, a compromise was made about having the sessions in school, but swapping the times and dates to ensure there was minimal disruption to the CYP's curriculum. In situations like this is maybe helpful to discuss with the school, (with the CYP's permission) to ascertain when the appointment can take place that will cause the least disruption.
- *Medication to be discussed at timely review of therapeutic intervention.* It was agreed that at the review of the evidence-based therapy, which is usually every five sessions, a conversation could be had about the use of medication. This compromise helped keep the parent or caregiver onside, knowing that it had not been forgotten, but also enables the CYP to have the evidence-based therapy they had requested. The discussion about medication does not mean that it will necessarily be prescribed, it would be hoped that the impact of the evidence-based therapy would be observable by all and medication may not needed at this point.
- *Parents/caregivers will be given a general update after each meeting.* It was agreed that a 5-min update will be given to parents in a very generalised way after each meeting. This again helped keep parents on side but allowed for privacy and empowered the CYP.

Whilst the above points offer an example of compromise, this could have been compromised differently. The importance is ensuring that both the CYP and the parent or caregiver are happy with the agreement. Using the circles of compromise demonstrates that the CYP and the parent or caregiver have been heard, listened to and validated, which are important attributes in establishing a compromise that will work for all parties. The circles of compromise are transferable to many different aspects of negotiation within many different settings.

11.12   Child Involvement and Participation Resources

There are a number of resources that can be helpful when working with CYP and families around consent. However, much of the work to enable a CYP to consent will include other subject areas and will not be about consent itself. For example, it might be concerning psycho-education around anxiety to inform the CYP about how anxiety works, then for them to understand the options of treatment in relation to treating or managing anxiety. Below are a number of resource hubs that span the mental health landscape that offer a range of worksheets, visual aids, information repositories and support for CYP and families.

www.minded.org.uk (Health Education England 2019) accompanies the CYP-IAPT strategy and offers training, advice and guidance for CYP, parents/caregivers and professionals. This website is also embedded within the e-learning for health website.

www.mycamhschoices.org (Anna Freud National Centre for Children and Families 2019) is developed by the Anna Freud Centre that includes information about a CYP's episode of care through CAMHS.

www.youngminds.org.uk (Young Minds 2019) is a resource from the UK's leading charity for child and adolescent mental health.

https://www.mhcirl.ie/File/htguidebook.pdf (Mental Health Commission 2009) is the headspace toolkit used for CYP that are an inpatient to help them be involved in decision-making and consent processes.

https://www.getselfhelp.co.uk/ (Vivyan 2018) offers information about disorders, diagnoses and intervention worksheets.

https://www.corc.uk.net/ (Child Outcome Research Consortium (CORC) 2019) supports the CYP-IAPT Routine Outcome Measures (ROM) in capturing patient outcomes, experience and feedback.

https://www.thecommunicationtrust.org.uk (The Communication Trust 2019) is an educational resource in supporting clinicians and parents in communicating with CYPs.

https://www.medicines.org.uk/emc/ (Datapharm 2019) is a medicine repository that has every medication in every dosage and form and gives information for professionals, CYPs and parents.

https://www.e-lfh.org.uk/ (Health Education England 2019) is the e-learning for health website that has a significant amount of resources to support nurses in a wide range of health environments.

This chapter has offered the key considerations when considering consent. This area of practice can be a very difficult area of CAMHS to navigate; if there are any difficulties in negotiating consent or supporting a CYP that the nurse struggles with, then supervision should be used as a constructive and supportive arena to progress the situation. There are numerous websites and resource hubs that can aid the nurse in developing their skills and knowledge base in involving the CYPs.

References

Abrines-Jaume N, Midgley N, Hopkins K, Hoffman J, Martin K, Law D, Wolpert M (2016) A qualitative analysis of implementing shared decision making in child and adolescent mental health services in the United Kingdom: stages and facilitators. Clin Child Psychol Psychiatry 21(1):19–31

Alderson P (2007) Competent children? Minors' consent to health care treatment and research. Soc Sci Med 65:2272–2283

Alderson P, Montgomery J (1996) Health care choices: making decisions with children. Institute for Public Policy Research, London

Al-Samsam RH (2008) Legal aspects of consent to treatment in children. Paediatr Child Health 18(10):469–473

Anna Freud National Centre for Children and Families (2019) On my mind/my CAMHS choices [online]. www.mycamhschoices.org. Accessed 31 Jan 2019

Billick SB, Edwards JL, Burgert W, Serlen JR, Bruni SM (1998) A clinical study of competency in child psychiatric inpatients. J Am Acad Psychiatry Law 26(4):587–594

Bolam v Friern Hospital Management Committee (1957) 1 WLR 582

Bolitho v City and Hackney Health Authority (1997) 3 W.L.R. 1151

Boyden J (2005) Childhood and the policy makers: a comparative perspective on the globalisation of childhood. In: James A, Prout A (eds) Constructing and reconstructing childhood: contemporary issues in the sociological study of childhood. Falmer Press, London, pp 218–221

Boylan J, Braye S (2006) Paid, professionalised and proceduralised: can legal and policy frameworks for child advocacy give voice to children and young people? J Soc Welf Fam Law 28(3–4):233–249

CAMHS EBPU (2014) Closing the gap through changing relationships final report for closing the gap through changing relationships (award holders). The Health Foundation, London

Cantwell B, Scott S (1995) Children's wishes, children's burdens. J Soc Welf Fam Law 17(3):337–354

Care Quality Commission (2017) Brief guide BG004: brief guide: capacity and competence in under 18s [online]. https://www.cqc.org.uk/sites/default/files/20180228_briefguide-capacity_consent_under_18s_v2.pdf. Accessed 13 Jan 2019

Child and Adolescent Mental Health Services (2008) Children and young people in mind: the final report of the national CAMHS review (the final report) [online]. http://webarchive.nationalarchives.gov.uk/20081230004520/publications.dcsf.gov.uk/eorderingdownload/camhs-review.pdf. Accessed 22 Nov 2018

Chitsabesan P (2018) The importance of engaging children and young people in the commissioning and delivery of mental health services [online]. https://www.england.nhs.uk/blog/the-importance-of-engaging-children-and-young-people-in-the-commissioning-and-delivery-of-mental-health-services/. Accessed 13 Jan 2019

CORC (2019) [Online]. https://www.corc.uk.net/. Accessed 31 Jan 2019

Cox AM, Brannigan C, Harling M, Townend M (2016) Factors that influence decision making by 8-12 year olds in child and adolescent mental health services (CAMHS): a systematic review. Res Policy Plan 31(3):195–207

Cox AM, Brannigan C, Harling M (2017) Recording and documenting consent of 8-12 year olds in an outpatient child and adolescent mental health service. Ment Health Pract 21(2):29–37

Data Protection Act (2018) Data protection act [online]. http://www.legislation.gov.uk/ukpga/2018/12/contents/enacted. Accessed 9 Nov 2018

Datapharm (2019) Electronic medicines compendium [online]. https://www.medicines.org.uk/emc/. Accessed 31 Jan 2019

Department of Health (2003) Getting the right start: NSF for children. Standard for hospital services [online]. https://www.gov.uk/government/uploads/system/uploads/attachment_data/file/199953/Getting_the_right_start_-_National_Service_Framework_for_Children_Standard_for_Hospital_Services.pdf. Accessed 22 Nov 2018

Department of Health (2009) Reference guide to consent for examination or treatment, 2nd edn. Department of Health, London

Dictionary.com (2018) Consent [online]. https://www.dictionary.com/browse/consent. Accessed 9 Nov 2018

Didcock EA (2007) Issues of consent and competency in children and young people. Paediatr Child Health 17(11):425–428

Donnelly C (2010) Reflections of a Guardian Ad Litem on the participation of looked after children on public law proceedings. Child Care Pract 16(2):181–193

European Parliament and the Council of the European Union (2016) GDPR regulations [online]. https://eur-lex.europa.eu/legal-content/EN/TXT/PDF/?uri=CELEX:32016R0679&from=EN. Accessed 9 Nov 2018

Gillick v Norfolk and Wisbech Health Authority (1985) 2 W.L.R. 413

Great Ormond Street Hospital for Children NHS Foundation Trust & The Common Room, 2019) Mefirst [online]. http://www.mefirst.org.uk/. Accessed 13 Jan 2019

Griffith R (2016) What is Gillick? Hum Vaccin Immunother 12(1):244–247

Health Education England (2019) E-learning for health/MIndEd [online]. https://www.e-lfh.org.uk/. Accessed 31 Jan 2019

Humanium (2010) Children's rights history [online]. https://www.humanium.org/en/childrens-rights-history/. Accessed 12 Nov 2018

Information Commissioners Office (2018) What do we need to consider when choosing a basis for processing children's personal data? [online]. https://ico.org.uk/for-organisations/guide-to-the-general-data-protection-regulation-gdpr/children-and-the-gdpr/what-do-we-need-to-consider-when-choosing-a-basis-for-processing-children-s-personal-data/. Accessed 9 Nov 2018

James A, Prout A (eds) (1997) Constructing and reconstructing childhood: new directions in the sociological study of childhood. Falmer, London

Jones P, Welch S (2010) Rethinking children's rights. Attitudes in contemporary society. Continuum International Publishing Group, London

Larcher V, Hutchinson A (2009) How should paediatricians assess Gillick competence? Arch Dis Child 95:307–311

MaClean A (2002) Beyond Bolam and Bolitho. Med Law Int 5(2):205–230

Mental Capacity Act (2005) Mental capacity act [online]. http://www.legislation.gov.uk/ukpga/2005/9/section/4. Accessed 12 Nov 2018

Mental Health Commission (2009) Headspace toolkit. For young people who are inpatients of mental health services [online]. https://www.mhcirl.ie/File/htguidebook.pdf. Accessed 31 Jan 2019

National Children's Bureau (2019) Building the participation of children and young people [online]. https://www.ncb.org.uk/what-we-do/our-priorities/sen-and-disability/projects-and-programmes/building-participation-children. Accessed 13 Jan 2019

NHS (2019) Fluoxetine [online]. https://www.nhs.uk/medicines/fluoxetine-prozac/. Accessed 13 Jan 2019

NHSE (2018) CYP-IAPT programme [online]. https://www.england.nhs.uk/mental-health/cyp/iapt/. Accessed 12 Nov 2018

NICE (2019) National Institute of Health and Care Excellence [online]. https://www.nice.org.uk/. Accessed 13 Jan 2019

NMC (2015) Code of conduct [online]. https://www.nmc.org.uk/standards/code/read-the-code-online/. Accessed 27 Jan 2019

Parekh SA (2006) Child consent and the law: an insight and discussion into the law relating to consent and competence. Child Care Health Dev 33(1):78–82

Paul M, Foreman DM, Kent L (2000) Outpatient clinic attendance and consent from children and young people: ethical perspectives and practical considerations. Clin Child Psychol Psychiatry 5(2):203–211

R v Bournewood Community & Mental Health NHS Trust (1997) 3 W.L.R. 107

Royal College of Gynaecologists (2016) The impact of the Montgomery ruling. Obstet Gynaecol Winter:20–21

Sidaway v Board of Governors of the Bethlem Royal Hospital (1985) A.C. 871

Simms v Simms (2003) 2 W.L.R. 1465

Tan JOA, Fegert JM (2004) Capacity and competence in child and adolescent psychiatry. Health Care Anal 12(4):285–294

Tan JOA, Passerini GE, Stewart A (2007) Consent and confidentiality in clinical work with young people. Clin Child Psychol Psychiatry 12(2):191–210

The Communication Trust (2019) [Online]. https://www.thecommunicationtrust.org.uk. Accessed 31 Jan 2019

UK Government (2018) Parental rights [online]. https://www.gov.uk/parental-rights-responsibilities/apply-for-parental-responsibility. Accessed 22 Nov 2018

Vivyan C (2018) Get self help [online]. https://www.getselfhelp.co.uk/index.html. Accessed 31 Jan 2019

Wellesley H, Jenkins I (2009) Consent in children. Anaesth Intensive Care Med 10(4):196–199

Wheeler R (2006) Gillick or Fraser? A plea for consistency over competence in children Gillick and Fraser are not interchangeable. Br Med J 332:807

Young Minds (2019) [Online]. www.youngminds.org.uk. Accessed 31 Jan 2019

Chapter 12
Summary

Laurence Baldwin

12.1 Reflections

Why is nursing important in helping with children and young people's mental health? At my interview for my first community CAMHS post I was asked, by a clinical psychologist, what I thought I would bring to the team by virtue of being a nurse? They had already asked what I might bring as an individual, so I was a little baffled, but I managed to get through the question, and got the job, but I can't honestly recall what I said. I do remember than thinking that it was a rather inadequate answer, and that I needed to discover what nurses did do in the community that was a *nursing* function. On the adolescent in-patient ward where I was working at the time, the essential 24/7 nursing care approach was fairly obvious, so I hadn't really thought about it in any depth. When I started the community job, the overlap between what the different disciplines brought to the task, the generic function of community CAMHS, made me wonder for a while if there as anything different about what we did. The only other CPN in the team, however, worked in a very similar manner to me, despite having trained in New Zealand, so I thought there must be something about that training and orientation that made us a bit different from the social worker (who became a systemic psychotherapist), the clinical psychologist, and the child and adolescent psychiatrist. As the team started to grow and include other disciplines, a couple more nurses, an art psychotherapist, another doctor, the feeling that there were some distinctive differences grew, but it was very difficult to articulate what those differences were, and whether they were because the nurses had something different to add to the mix from their nurse training.

For a while I felt that the idea that nurses have an eclectic approach and were essentially the glue that held other teams together had a lot going for it as the answer. This was based on observations about what jobs nurses did that others were reluctant

L. Baldwin (✉)
School of Nursing, Midwifery and Health, Coventry University, Coventry, Warwickshire, UK
e-mail: ac1273@coventry.ac.uk

© Springer Nature Switzerland AG 2020

193

L. Baldwin (ed.), *Nursing Skills for Children and Young People's Mental Health*,
https://doi.org/10.1007/978-3-030-18679-1_12

to do, because their vision of what their role entailed were much better defined. Some of this became more obvious at critical times, when I noticed, rather flippantly, I admit, that it was always the nurses who put up the Christmas tree and decorated the waiting room. It's difficult to speculate on why this happened without offending colleagues that I admire and respect, but there was something about the nursing approach which made us feel we had to create the right atmosphere for families when they arrived, whilst others did not see this as quite so important. One year we refused to do it and it was a miserable atmosphere in the waiting room! I later discarded this theory anyway when I worked elsewhere and the reception staff were the ones who did the Christmas decorations. But it did make me notice other things that some professions did which seemed 'wrong' to me, but were part of the 'taken for granted' element of professions. Doctors are happy to have 'Thank You' cards up on their walls, and wear smart suit and tie, or more formal styles of clothing for the female doctors, whilst nurses tend more to wear 'smart casual' (I never wore a tie, unless I was going to a management meeting!). This seems to reflect the expert position which the medical profession takes, and which the public expects of them. Clinical psychologists seemed much more wedded to specific models and attached a lot of importance to maintaining fidelity to those models, and the social worker was much more aware of child protection issues and social models of care. All of them, however, also had engagement skills and developed therapeutic relationships with the children and young people, and their families, which I thought was what nursing was about, but they didn't attach as much importance to this as the nurses did, and maybe spent less time on those aspects because they also had core philosophies from their professions which had primacy, and added on the 'people skills' parts.

In terms of professional identity I learnt that defining yourself by what you don't do—as my colleagues were doing, and which as nurses we often do, at the time we didn't prescribe, we couldn't perform some reserved psychologist's assessments, and we didn't diagnose—is called 'othering' (Davies 2003) and is a rather negative way of defining yourself. It is most classically expressed in the studies which look at how nurses and doctors interact, the 'Doctor-Nurse game' (Stein et al. 1990). As expended roles have developed the list of things that nurses don't do has reduced—I took the independent prescribing course much later in my career, for example, so that also affects what defines the difference between nurses and medical doctors. As I wrote up and presented my early thoughts (Limerick and Baldwin 2000; Baldwin 2002), people started to ask me what was the answer to the questions I was asking them, and I still didn't have a good answer. The difficulty in verbalizing things continued, mostly because many of my colleagues who were from different professions also exhibited the skills which I saw as essential to nursing. Through a rather in-depth process of study (Baldwin 2008) I came to think that the skills we have looked at in this book were not something which were exclusive to nursing, but which were the ones which, as nurses, our underlying philosophy and training put the most emphasis on. In fact, very few things are exclusive to one professional group in mental health teams, and CAMHS teams in particular, and hanging your identity on those things which only you can do is also a rather precarious position to take. Much of the exclusive parts of medical profession, prescribing, diagnosis and application of certain parts of the Mental Health Act, have been eroded and can now be performed by other professions, which allows some managers to question the need for how many of them we need, or to fill positions with other staff when there are shortages. Many of the clinical psychologists I have worked with have been very reluctant to be pigeon-holed with performing the copyrighted assessments that others cannot do. At the same time other professional groups, clinical psychologists, psychotherapists and medical doctors still put time and effort into maintaining a clear professional identity, and being clear about why it is important that they are part of the team. Nursing has always been reluctant to spend too much time on this and has continued to struggle to define what it does.

12.2   Is There a Unique Contribution That Nursing Brings?

Nursing is both simple and complex, and the best nurses (as with every profession) make the complex task that they perform look effortless and natural. This brings with it two main difficulties, firstly that other people may think that it is *just* a simple task, one that can be done by anyone, perhaps even without much training, even 'intuitively'. The second problem is that explaining, or verbalizing the complexities of an apparently simple task becomes more difficult, to the point that some people seem to be so much part of their role that they forget that what they are doing is complex, and that they 'take for granted' what they do, maybe even assume that others would do the work in the same way. The famous oil well firefighter Red Adair allegedly said: 'If you think getting a professional to do a job is expensive, try getting an amateur'. Whilst his area of expertise was more explosive, nursing, even child mental health nursing, deals with life and death situations, and can potentially have fatal outcomes, or long-standing poor health outcomes if not done well.

We are working in a time when the pressures to provide quick and effective answers to complex problems, using often the cheapest measures, are enormous. In nursing in general work has been done to look at staffing and skill mix, with an increasing amount of evidence that the best care (and the best outcomes in terms of lowering mortality, how many patients actually live and die) is provided when levels of qualified staff are higher. Although most of this work has been done on acute medical wards (Griffiths et al. 2018), the principles must surely be same when looking at an equally complex area of children and young people's mental health. Professor Alison Leary recently commented (Leary and Punshon 2019) that the weight of evidence is not actually affecting policy as well as one might hope in a sector where high value is put on following an evidence base. She noted that nursing is arguably one of those areas which is only noticed in its absence, or when something goes wrong, as in the Mid-Staffordshire tragedy. Whilst this study concentrates on acute nurse staffing and safety, the authors note in their conclusions that they found no real examination of the impact of numbers in a 'knowledge intense' profession and speculated that the complexity of the nursing role makes it difficult to define.

This is in somewhat stark contrast to other professional groups, who are much better at defining what is their exclusive domain and what others cannot do, to the extent of protecting it by law. In the UK, 'registered nurse' is a protected title and cannot be used by anyone who is not on the NMC register, but the title 'nurse' is widely used by a range of different jobs. There remain a few areas where legally a nurse *is* required, medication management, for example, and curiously the 'Named Nurse' role in Safeguarding Children. It remains harder to define within CAMHS what only nurses can do, the expanded role of independent nurse prescribing being an exception.

Within the therapies the different psychotherapies have been much better at defining their unique contributions to the field, and defining what constitutes a 'qualified psychotherapist' within their area of expertise. Both cognitive behavioural and systemic psychotherapy, for example, now insist that you cannot call yourself a cognitive behavioural psychotherapist or systemic psychotherapist unless you are trained at Masters level and registered with the British Association for Counselling and Psychotherapy (BACP). The BACP is not a state registering body, like the NMC, HCPC or GMC, but does regulate the psychotherapies at a technically lower level. Whilst many CAMH nurses have been able to access additional training in CBT and systemic psychotherapies via the CYP-IAPT programme, those trainings are focused at delivering skills for a function, and not at Masters level, so nurses are not accessing full qualification through that programme. This process of protecting knowledge is an interesting one in terms of professional identity and how we see ourselves. In the early days of family therapy (before it insisted on calling itself systemic psychotherapy), the techniques of systems thinking and their alliance with nursing's tendency to holism meant that some nurse theorists saw this as a fruitful area for development. Shirley Smoyak, writing from an American perspective (1975), described nurses as family therapists, and Wright and Leahey (2008) developed their family nursing model based on structural family therapy as we have seen, though they never refer to nurses as family therapists. Whilst this can be seen as a natural form of protectionism, cognitive behavioural therapies followed a similar route in determining exclusivity by virtue of training which ensures fidelity to the theoretical model, and it does pose the question of whether nurses who train in those therapies lose their nursing identity and instead become therapists. Similar issues exist for social workers and allied health professionals who train in the psychotherapies, and my conclusions over the years have been that the strength of the underlying conceptual base for your identity (Baldwin 2008) determines whether you continue to see yourself primarily as a nurse after fully training as a psychotherapist, or whether that conceptual base takes over your thinking and you think of yourself as primarily a psychotherapist, rather than a nurse (or social worker or AHP).

12.3 Professional Identity and Nursing Strengths in CAMH Nursing

As we have seen throughout this volume there is a strong attachment to the identity of nursing, but rather more difficulty in adequately defining what nurses bring, and what the conceptual basis of nursing brings of value to CAMH. Primarily my colleagues and I have drawn on the mental health nursing concepts of interpersonal relations, the concepts of therapeutic relationships, and therapeutic use of self that were promoted by Hildegard Peplau and consequently by Altschul and Barker, in the UK. However, CAMH nurses also come from other fields, children and young people's nursing and learning disabilities nursing, where this tradition is not so strongly emphasized, so using this as a unique feature has become problematic. Consequently I have tended to use the idea that rather than having uniqueness nursing brings strengths which it prioritises or 'privileges' as being more important than other professional groups do. They tend to use these areas too, but they are not core to the thinking—defining them exactly is tricky, though I tried to outline them in Chap. 1, and Marie Armstrong uses a slightly different (but broadly similar) set of skills, whilst Gemma Robbins and Steph Sargeant give a slightly different slant from a children's nurse perspective.

Just because it is complicated or difficult to define doesn't mean we shouldn't continue to attempt to define what we bring. Many people claim to have an eclectic toolbox of skills they use in their work with children and young people, but the importance of this is knowing what each tool is and when to use it. Katrina Singhatey and Moira Goodman showed in their chapter that their emphasis on putting themselves alongside the people they worked with didn't stop them from using both CBT and systemic tools when they were useful, but they did so consciously. Annie Cox likewise draws out the differences and similarities of different approaches to therapy, and shows how nurses can ensure that the important issue of children and young people understanding what they are being asked to consent to is addressed thoroughly.

The central thesis of this book has been to try and unpick some of the nursing skills that we use, often referred to as 'soft skills' because they are hard to define, and often they are so embedded in our thinking that we take for granted the way in which we work. The idea that actually these very qualities are actually exactly what children and young people need is borne out by Leanne Walker's conversations with Hannah and Danni, and reflected in the wider participation work that Leanne has been involved in nationally and internationally. Of course children and young people also need people who can diagnose carefully and draw on expert knowledge, and they need people who are highly trained in models of therapy and care which are proven to work, but that they say they most need are simple things like people who care enough to spend time with them, listen to their stories, believe in them as individuals and stick with them through the most difficult parts of their journey. Nurses have those qualities at the heart of what they do, and should be valued or what they bring, even if they aren't very good at explaining what or why they are doing it.

References

Baldwin L (2002) The nursing role in out-patient child and adolescent mental health services. J Clin Nurs 11:520–525

Baldwin L (2008) The discourse of professional identity in child and adolescent mental health services. PhD thesis, University of Nottingham. Access from the University of Nottingham repository http://eprints.nottingham.ac.uk/10504/1/LBaldwinThesis2008.pdf

Davies C (2003) Workers, professions and identity. In: Henderson J, Atkinson D (eds) Managing care in context. Routledge/Open University Press, London

Griffiths P, Maruotti L, Saucedo AR, Redfern OC, Ball JE, Briggs J, Dall'Ora C, Schmidt PE, Smith JB (2018) Nurse staffing, nursing assistants and hospital mortality: retrospective longitudinal cohort study. BMJ Qual Saf. https://doi.org/10.1136/bmjqs-2018-008043. Accessed 26 Apr 2019

Leary A, Punshon G (2019) Determining acute nurse staffing: a hermeneutic review of an evolving science. BMJ Open 9(3):e025654. https://doi.org/10.1136/bmjopen-2018-025654. Accessed 26 Apr 2019

Limerick M, Baldwin L (2000) Nursing in outpatient child and adolescent mental health. Nurs Stand 15(13–15):43–45

Stein L, Watts DT, Howell T (1990) The doctor nurse game revisited. Nurs Outlook 38:264–268

Wright LM, Leahey M (2008) Nurse and families: a guide to assessment and intervention, 5th edn. F.A. Davies Company, Philadelphia, PA

The manufacturer's authorised representative in the EU is Springer
Nature Customer Service Centre GmbH, Europaplatz 3, 69115 Heidelberg,
Germany. If you have any concerns regarding our products, please
contact ProductSafety@springernature.com

Printed and bound by CPI Group (UK) Ltd, Croydon, CR0 4YY
23/04/2026
02095604-0004